T

His   ;

The Art of History Taking

Kashinath Padhiary

MD FICP

Associated Professor of Medicine

SCB Medical College

Cuttack

JAYPEE BROTHERS
MEDICAL PUBLISHERS (P) LTD
New Delhi

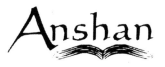

Tunbridge Wells
UK

First published in the UK by

Anshan Ltd
in 2005
6 Newlands Road
Tunbridge Wells
Kent TN4 9AT, UK

Tel/Fax: +44 (0)1892 557767
E-mail: info@anshan.co.uk
www.anshan.co.uk

ISBN 1 904798 314

British Library Cataloguing in Publication Data
A catalogue record for this book is available from the British Library

Printed in India by Sanat Printers, Kundli.

To my students

Dear students
Nobody can teach you
    Unless you try to learn,
A teacher cannot teach you
    He can expose your ignorance only,
Don't expect too much from a teacher
    Because his knowledge is limited,
Rather, try to learn from the books
    Under the guidance of your teacher,
Never compromise quality in learning
    As the future (treating and teaching) will be in your hand,
We may not be excellent
    But we all have a scope to excel.

Preface

Is there a need for such a book?

With the progress of scientific knowledge more and more investigative procedures are available. These investigations have helped to reach at a more complete diagnosis, but simultaneously have increased the total cost of therapy. It is my observation that younger generations of doctors are becoming more and more dependent on these investigations. Investigations always do not give clear picture; at times confusing information is obtained particularly in a country like India where standardized laboratories are very few. These young doctors do not realize how much information can be obtained from a well taken history and how it can limit the number of investigations; thereby reducing the cost of therapy. Worldwide it has been felt that there is an absolute need to reduce the cost of therapy. I have tried to explain the amount of information we can get from history in few important systems; but importance of history is very much there in each and every case, medical, surgical or gynaecological or in other fields.

It is my observation over the years that undergraduate students take a bizarre history. Postgraduate students also take history without knowing the importance of every aspect of the history. Often teachers just tell the students to collect the history without teaching them how to take the history, nor guide them while they are taking history. In view of PG students coming from several parts of the country and enquiring from them, I have noticed that this is the practice more or less everywhere. In fact, I have seen teachers giving undue importance to physical examination and investigations. None of the commonly available books of clinical methods describe the intricacies of history taking. The pages covered for history taking in these books is much less in comparison to the pages covered for physical examination. When the same thing is repeated at bedside, students fail to realize the importance of history. At times confusing things happen. For example, in history of present illness, no leading questions should be asked, but in practice almost all physicians ask leading questions. A beginner gets confused by that. Similarly, chief complaints are supposed to be recorded in patient's own language, but often the language the patient uses is not understood well, nor there is a scientific counterpart available in the books. So the information collected do not serve any purpose.

There are several other points which need clarifications. I shall try to discuss these points so that the students will be able to collect a fairly informative history. This book cannot teach the total aspects of history taking. Once the students realize the importance of history, they can take better history than I can describe or anybody can teach. I hope this book will be of use to all the students of medicine.

Kashinath Padhiary

Contents

Contents

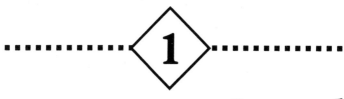

General Considerations

> Uncommon manifestations of common diseases are more common than common manifestations of uncommon diseases.

Reaching at the Diagnosis

It is an age old saying that diagnosis should precede treatment. To decide that somebody is suffering from a disease or not, it needs evaluations of all aspects of diagnostic principles. These principles are:

1. History taking
2. General physical examination
3. Systemic examination
4. Investigations.

Each step has got significance. In some cases history alone may be enough, in some cases systemic examination may yield the maximum information and in the other cases it may be required to ask for a series of investigations. As one proceeds from history onwards, one should assess how nearer he has come to the diagnosis at the end of every step. By proceeding this way one can narrow down the differential diagnosis; hence, one can logically plan the line of investigations. Proper planning of investigations is very much required as some of the investigations are costly and some are risky. Over the years clinical diagnosis has been found to be the most cost-effective step in reaching at the diagnosis and it can be utilized anywhere, can be repeated several times. Investigations are not always productive. At times unreliable, at times ambiguous, as there are very few standardized laboratories in a country like India. Whether to accept a report or not, needs detail knowledge of the clinical situation. So one should always try to acquire as much clinical skill as possible. In fact, it has been advised that "no doctor should request any special investigation unless he knows what information relevant to the problem it is likely to provide, and has some idea of its cost and of its possible danger to the patient" (Hutchison, 18th edn, Page 4)

Importance of History Taking

With the progress of time, diagnosis of human disease has become easier due to availability of several investigative facilities like X-ray, ultrasound, echocardiography, CT scan, MRI scan and others. However, the value of clinical diagnosis has not decreased. All the investigations are supplementary to the clinical diagnosis only. History contributes the major part to the clinical diagnosis.

In the history taking we evaluate the feelings of a person. There is no machine to measure or assess the feeling of a man. At times it becomes difficult for a person to express his feelings in words, sometimes he expresses in gestures and these gestures often give important clues to diagnosis.

The physical examination and the investigations reveal the changes present at the time of examination, does not tell anything about the temporal profile of the illness. But, it is the temporal profile of the illness which is most often required to clinch the diagnosis. This is only brought out by a thorough history taking. Even a probable diagnosis can be known about an illness which occurred years back by detail analysis of symptoms. This importance of history in clinical diagnosis must have been realized by all physicians in their lifetime. However, I want to quote one statement from a leading book on clinical method, Hutchison's clinical method, 20th edition:

"Remember that the examination can only reveal abnormalities present at the time of the examination. The history, on the other hand can reveal aspects of the temporal development of the illness. The history and examinations are thus complementary, but often the history is more important."

In a neurological case one should be able to give three-fourth of the diagnosis at the end of the history taking. If this has not been achieved, history taking is told to be inadequate (Bickerstaff, 6th edn, 1996; Page 8). The same author has also stated: *'No one can expect to go through his career and to be right all the time, but most error arise from inadequate taking of history and inadequate physical examination—particularly the inadequate history.'*

It is equally important in a respiratory case also. I have felt that history gives more information in a respiratory case than in a neurological case. Physical findings are often confusing and unreliable. In relation to history in respiratory case, Hutchison states: *As with every aspect of diagnosis in medicine, the key to success is a clear and carefully recorded history* (20th edn, 1995; Page 141). Another leading author on respiratory diseases, GK Crofton states. '*In many instances careful history taking is more important than elicitation of elegant, but possibly misleading physical signs*'(The respiratory system, Macleod's clinical examination, 9th edn, 1995; page 136). The clinical history and examination are fundamental to assessment of respiratory health even in the epoch of computer-assisted tomography and broncho-alveolar lavage. In deed too great an emphasis on the technology of medicine may lead to atrophy of clinical study and thus a loss of judgment in the assessment of an individual's health(The clinical manifestations of respiratory diseases, Crofton and Douglas's Respiratory Diseases; A Seaton, D Seaton, AG Leitech, 4th edn,1989; Page104).

In diseases of the Gastrointestinal system too history is equally important. Little information will be obtained by examination of these patients. Pain is a common symptom of intra-abdominal diseases. In patient with abdominal pain, detail interrogation and clinical judgment is essential before investigations are performed. If this is neglected, unnecessary tests may result in the discovery of asymptomatic abnormalities, such as hiatus hernia or gallstones, leading to inappropriate management and even unnecessary surgery.

(The alimentary and genitourinary systems, MJ Ford, DW Haner Hodges; Macleod's clinical Examination, 9th edn, 1995; Page 162).

From these Quotes from different renowned authors and from the experiences of my colleagues and from my own, I can conclude that in every case history taking is of utmost importance to reach at a diagnosis and for proper planning of investigation and treatment. I shall again re-emphasize the value of history taking in individual chapters.

History Taking—An Art

History taking is basically a process of understanding the feeling of an individual. These feelings are nothing but the symptoms of different diseases. Feelings cannot be quantitated, so cannot be always expressed in scientific terms, nor can be satisfactorily expressed in words. Scientific understanding of a disease is nothing but understanding the bodily changes in terms of changes in anatomy and physiology. History taking not only tries to assess the bodily changes but also its affect on mind. So, while taking history, look for the affect of the illness on the mind in addition to its affect on the body. This can be done by looking for the nonverbal communications and the body language. In fact, there may not be any physical ailment at all, yet the patient becomes symptomatic and the significance of these symptoms can be known from the body language. How to study the body language and the emotional aspect of an illness cannot be taught theoretically, hence, this has to be learnt by seeing patients under guidance; so this becomes an art.

To take a good history, one has to go down to the level of the thinking of the patient. The words the lay man uses, one has to understand clearly what he means by that. One has to know the exact nature of the work of the patient and how the illness affects his day-to-day work. Understanding the language of the patient is mandatory for correct assessment of the history. This is particularly true for a country like India, where people use several languages. Even in the same language there are several colloquial words and terms which are also to be understood clearly. Whenever required the help of a good interpreter should be taken.

Because history taking is basically a mode of conversation, so the doctor should encourage the patient to speak freely without any reservation. An environment for free talk should be created. You have to ensure him that you also feel for his illness and you are there to help him. Remember that while you are taking history the patient also marks how attentively you are listening to him. If you show dissatisfaction or displeasure repeatedly, he does not feel like talking and may give a confusing history. Similarly if your attention is diverted frequently to other things while listening to the patient's complaints, he feels that you are neither interested nor attentive to his problem. Due to this type of attitude, patients lose faith in the doctor even if he has diagnosed and treated correctly. I remember a father took his young son to a renowned physician. The consultant wrote the age of the child to be one and half years instead of one and half months and accordingly prescribed the drugs. This was noted by the father after coming out of the consultation chamber.

He returned back and pointed it to the doctor, but the doctor did not take it seriously. The father lost faith in the doctor and did not follow the prescription. The father had also marked that while the doctor was taking history of his child he was often talking to others. This example speaks that patients do notice how attentive you are to them. So, while consultation is being done too many outsiders should not be allowed. This will make the patient nervous, likely to divert the attention of the doctor and the patient will not feel free to speak, particularly matters related to sex and personal life.

Like any other art, practice makes a man perfect, so also in the art of history taking one has to practice daily to improve. More one feels for the patient, more one gets involved with the patient and more one can extract the information from the patient.

Often people do not know what to tell before a doctor and do not understand which part of the history is to be elaborated. This is either due to illiteracy or due to nervousness. Whatever may be the reason it is the duty of the doctor to collect a reliable history. To eradicate the initial anxiety and nervousness from the patient's mind try to greet the patient by name whenever possible. Try to discuss topics unrelated to his ailment. Like commenting on the dress, asking about his children in case of elderly people, school and education in case of school-going children. At times these discussions can reveal key points. If the patient is giving the unnecessary details of a minor point, instead of getting irritated on him, listen to him patiently and simultaneously ask the details of the points which you feel to be important. Often patients try to speak medical terms without knowing their significance and meaning. They should be dissuaded from this. At times patients tell more about their treatment than about their illness. This should be discouraged also. Also there are patients who show several consultation papers without telling much about their illness. Tell them to show the papers at the end of the consultation, because these papers are likely to misguide the examiner. However, these papers have their own importance which will be discussed later. I always recommend students to evaluate the cases independently so that they can assess themselves after going through the papers of experienced consultants.

Never show dissatisfaction or displeasure in words or in action while listening to the patient. For example, if a patient passes urine or vomits before you, remain quite, ask the attendant to clean the patient and the room, ask the patient to relax on a bed for some time and then discuss or examine him later. Similarly, if there is a foul smelling ulcer or foul breath, do not sniff or spit before the patient. These cases are often discarded by the family members and friends; their only hope is the doctor, that he will be able to do something to get rid of his problem, so that he will be able to go back to social life. Instead, if he feels that the doctor also dislikes him, he may not feel like living and may attempt to commit suicide.

The doctor is in an advantageous position; rather he is in a better position than other relatives including parents to know the facts about the patient. The facts which are not told to the relatives may be revealed to the doctor. Grown up children will not like to undress before their parents, but will not hesitate to do so before the doctor. That the doctor is in an advantageous position, he should not take its undue advantage. One has to maintain the privacy of every patient and the secrecy of facts revealed to him should be maintained. It is a common experience that often doctors become good friends of many patients, particularly elderly people. These people often express unnecessary details of their family matters.

Sequence of History Taking

Traditionally after collecting biodata, which includes age, sex, religion, address, occupation; the chief complain, history of present illness, history of past illness, family history, personal history, menstrual and obstetrics history and treatment history are to be taken. However, this scheme need not be strictly followed while applying on an individual case. In fact, some authors recommend taking past history and family history earlier than the present illness. This helps to understand the person and his illness more completely and more clearly. I personally agree with this recommendation. I am giving two examples here how this is helpful.

Suppose, a case of rheumatic heart disease complains of fever for fifteen days and gives history of dental extraction twenty days back. Here fever is the present illness and tooth extraction comes under the past illness. If this case is presented in a sequence like – a case of known rheumatic heart disease had tooth extraction twenty days back and having fever for fifteen days, it appears that this patient is suffering from infective endocarditis.

Similarly, if a woman comes with unconsciousness and is pregnant also, it is better to tell from the beginning that 'a pregnant lady coming with loss of consciousness for so many days duration'. Here one need not wait for obstetric history to mention about her being pregnant. Presenting this way will make the clinical situation clearer.

It is not important in what order history is collected provided one does not miss any point and the examiner has been able to understand every aspect of the history. In fact, in nervous patients it is wiser to discuss his personal life earlier than about his illness, so that the patient gains confidence and tells the history clearly. However, for beginners it is better to stick to the sequence, so that they will not miss any point. Similarly in critically ill patients few points from history should be collected and no delay should be made to institute the first aid to save the life of the patient. Once the condition of the patient is stabilized details of the history can be collected. One should not waste time in getting unnecessary details of the history when the patient is in a gasping state. Here are the situations where treatment precedes the diagnosis, though in most other situations diagnosis should precede treatment. I have seen students taking history from the relatives while the patient is already dead.

The Leading Question

Ideally patients should be asked to narrate their story in their own words. Leading questions are not to be asked. Leading question is that which suggests its answer, usually as yes or no. But many patients do not give a cohesive history. These patients require asking some direct questions, often as leading questions. The physician has to be very careful in accepting the answers to leading questions. These answers should be cross verified, about their reliability. Because, often the patient replies in yes, to emphasize his complaints and replies in no if he wants to hide some points. In fact, some authors say that the best physician is he who can interpret the leading questions.

From whom History to be Collected

Under ordinary situations patient himself should be asked to tell the history. Often relatives of the patient try to interfere in history collection. This should be discouraged. Even the most uneducated patient can tell about his illness with a little guidance from the doctor.

In case of a child, history should be collected from the parents, preferably from the mother. If detail of the illnesses of childhood is required, this can be collected from the parents or from any other senior family member who knows about his childhood.

In unconscious patients history should be collected from the persons who were present during the onset of the illness (often this gives clue points to diagnosis). He may be family member, room mate, class mate, colleague or teacher.

Similarly in patients with transient loss of consciousness like epilepsy or transient ischemic attack history should be collected from an eyewitness. Mentally retarded, deaf and dumb person's history should be collected from the people who ordinarily take their care. Because, they can notice the slightest changes in their activity or notice the symptoms of illness at the earliest.

Observing for Nonverbal Communications

While the patient is telling the story, observe the patient closely. The words he uses, the emotional attachment to the words, movement of hands and other body parts, etc. should be marked.

For example, while describing the anginal pain the patient may start weeping, which signifies the severity of pain. Simultaneously if he is moving his hands over the sternum, implying that the pain is retrosternal in site. If the patient is moving his hand over a wide area on the abdominal wall while describing abdominal pain, it is likely that the pain is not localized. If he points the site of pain with a finger, it is a localized pain as seen in pleurisy. If a patient is groaning with abdominal pain likely that it is a colicky pain. If a patient comes with a cloth tied over the head or on the abdomen very likely he is having headache or colicky abdominal pain respectively. If a patient is talking in a loud voice he is either nervous or deaf. If a patient is talking in a low voice, often looking at this side or the other, probably wants to speak something about sexual problem. If a patient is wearing a warm dress in summer season likely that he is having a chilly sensation (possibly due to fever). If a patient is not able to complete a sentence in one breath his vital capacity is low. If the patient is giving extensive details of his illness and treatment is likely to be a hypochondriac. At times patients produce a list of complaints often as many as ten to fifteen of them. It may be so that, none is genuine, suggesting that they are hypochondriac too. A patient of polyuria may come with a bucket of water with him because excessive thirst and non-availability of safe drinking water on the way. If a patient comes with a stick, it is likely that he is not sure of his stance or gait (either due to weakness or due to ataxia).

Chronic bodily illness often puts its impact on the mind. These patients move from doctor to doctor and if still don't get relief; they get depressed (thinking that they are suffering from an incurable disease). The depressed mood can be noted from their face and from their mode of talk. Likewise there are many more things which can be observed while taking history.

2

Personal Information

> *Be a man first then the doctor.*
> *See the man first then the disease.*
> *Don't miss the forest for a tree.*

Before collecting details of the ailments one should collect certain personal information like age, sex, locality, occupations, etc. At times these points hold the key to reach at a diagnosis.

AGE

Of several variables age is the singlemost point contributing to causation of diseases. Aging is inevitable, so also the age-related problems. Problems in elderly individuals are dementia, osteoarthritis, coronary artery disease (CAD), blindness due to cataract and so on. Chances of developing various types of malignancies increase with increase in age, but some cancers like chronic lymphatic leukaemia, multiple myeloma are mostly seen in elderly individuals only.

Many of the diseases found in old age may be primarily due to aging. Similar diseases if encountered in younger age there could be some specific precipitating factors/ risk factors. For example, a person of seventy years may suffer from CAD without having any risk factors, but if the same illness is encountered in a 40-year-old individual there could be some risk factors like smoking, hypertension, etc. Similarly if an elderly person presents with cerebrovascular disease it may be due to atherothrombosis; but if it is seen in a young person it may be due to cerebral embolism due to coexistence of rheumatic heart disease like mitral stenosis.

Some problems are common to children. Most of the congenital conditions are commonly encountered in childhood, at times very early in childhood. However, there are few congenital conditions which can manifest for the first time in adult life like coarctation of aorta, bicuspid aortic valve, rupture of Berry aneurism leading to subarachnoid haemorrhage and so on. Inborn errors of metabolism may present from early childhood. Excluding the congenital disorders; other conditions which are common to childhood, are poliomyelitis, diphtheria, whooping cough, measles, etc. Nutritional deficiency conditions are also common to childhood as their requirement per kg body weight is more. Kwashiorkor, Marasmus, and Vitamin A deficiency states are common in children. Overall malignancies are uncommon in children, but some malignancies are more frequently encountered in children like Wilms' tumor of kidney, acute lymphatic leukaemia, retinoblastoma, craniopharyngioma, medulloblastoma. Other common problems in children are foreign body in nose, ear or in the respiratory tract.

A child presenting with bleeding per anum might be suffering from rectal polyp and the same complaint in an elderly person may be due to carcinoma rectum. Acute rheumatic fever is more common in children so also Friedreich's ataxia. Both the conditions are seen in children of 5 to 15 years age group.

These are just few examples where age helps in making a diagnosis. But there are innumerable conditions where age plays a significant role in causation of the disease. Age is not only required for making a diagnosis, is also required for prescribing certain drugs. Digitalis is better tolerated by children than adults. Tetracycline can cause permanent staining of the teeth in children, quinolones can retard bone growth in children, opium alkaloids can cause marked constipation in elderly individuals, glucocorticosteroids for a long period in children can cause retardation of bone growth and the same in elderly individuals can cause pathological fractures.

Course of certain diseases also vary with age. For example, idiopathic thrombocytopenic purpura in children carries better prognosis than in adults. Nephrotic syndrome in children responds to steroids better than nephrotic syndrome occurring in adults.

SEX

Sex is also an important factor towards the causation of disease. As such diseases of the reproductive system will be found in the respective sex. Besides these, some diseases are more frequently encountered in females. Most of the endocrine disorders like Sheehan's syndrome, Addison's disease, Cushing's syndrome, thyrotoxicosis, hypothyroidism are more common in women. Rheumatoid arthritis, SLE and other collagen diseases are also more common in females. Bronchial adenomas, Primary pulmonary hypertension, Sydenham's chorea are also more common in females. Diseases which are transmitted as X-linked recessive mode are seen in males. Some such examples are haemophilias, G6 PD deficiency, red green colour blindness, Gout due to deficiency of HGPRT enzyme, Duchenne type muscular dystrophy. In a country like India smoking and alcoholism are mostly seen in males; hence, smoking and alcohol-related diseases are more common in males. Diseases like multiple myeloma are more common in males.

LOCALITY

There are several diseases which are peculiarly seen more frequently in certain geographical areas. This may be due to the environmental factors, genetic constitution of the people, certain practices peculiar to the place. Chagas' disease is seen in South American countries like Brazil, Argentina, Uruguay, Paraguay and Chile. Sleeping sickness is seen in Central and West African countries. Thalassaemia is common in Mediterranean countries, though there are pockets in other countries too. Multiple sclerosis and subacute combined degeneration of the cord, pernicious anaemia are common in temperate climate. Various types of encephalitis are also seen in specified geographical areas. Carcinoma stomach is more common amongst Japanese though coronary artery disease is less amongst them. Khangri cancer is common in Kashmir due to the habit of keeping a burning pot at abdomen. In India Goiter is common in Sub-Himalayan areas (Jammu and Kashmir, Punjab, Himachal Pradesh, Delhi, Uttar Pradesh, Bihar and West Bengal). This region is considered as the largest goiter belt in the world. This is due to less content of iodine in the water. Fluorosis is seen in certain places of Andhra Pradesh (Prakasam, Nalgonda, Nellore districts), Punjab, Haryana, Karnataka and Tamil Nadu. Kala azar is seen in states like Bihar and parts of West Bengal. Dracunculosis is seen in Rajasthan where people use step wells. Most of the helminthic infestations and other water-borne diseases are common in those countries (developing countries) where disposal of faeces is not proper and safe drinking water is not guaranteed. Bancroftian filariasis is more common in the coastal regions of Orissa, Andhra Pradesh, Tamil Nadu, Kerala and Gujarat. In those areas where vaccination is not widely done diseases like poliomyelitis and tetanus do occur. Certain diseases are not seen at certain places like Rabies is not seen in Australia, New Zealand and Japan; Yellow fever is not seen in India.

OCCUPATION

In addition to the above personal information occupation of the person at times contributes to the causation of ailments. While collecting occupation one should ask in detail about the exact nature of the work. Various types of Pneumoconiosis are by far the most common type of occupational disorders. Silicosis (silicon dusts) is seen in workers in sand blasting, metal grinding, ceramic industry, building and construction works, etc., anthracosis (Coal workers), asbestosis (Asbestos workers), byssinosis (Textile workers) are some of the examples. Persons taking care of animals (veterinarians) are more likely to suffer from Brucellosis. People carrying animal skins on their back are more likely to suffer Anthrax. Sewerage workers are more likely to suffer from Leptospirosis. Lead toxicity is seen in people working in lead industries. People exposed to chemicals like benzene may suffer from hypoplastic anaemia. Prolonged exposure to ionizing radiation and other types of radiations like X-rays can cause hypoplastic anaemia/ leukaemia. Non- vaccinated farmers and gardeners are more likely to suffer from tetanus. Bird handlers suffer more often from psittacosis and ornithosis. There are many more conditions related to occupation. In relation to occupation one should enquire about the present as well as past occupation and their duration.

3

Chief Complaints and Present Illness

> With the observations of thousands of our
> colleagues the knowledge has reached this state.
> Don't allow the power of observation to decline.

Chief complaints are the complaints which bring the patient
for medical help. Often this will give a guide to the diagnosis.
However, always it may not be possible to understand the
complaints. Here one can suggest a few words or phrases
to the patient so that it becomes scientifically meaningful.
All complaints should be recorded chronologically. Because,
all the symptoms may be the manifestations of one illness
at different stages or one may be related to the other as a
cause and effect. Ordinarily, the patient complains of that
which he thinks to be important. But for the purpose of
diagnosis this may not be true. For example: a patient may
come for haemoptysis (say for 2 days), but he fails to tell
that he was having cough for two months. Here the patient
deliberately does not do this. He does not understand that
both may be related. He complains of haemoptysis because

he feels it is an alarming symptom. If haemoptysis would not have occurred, he would not have come for medical help. For the doctor the chief complaints will be:

Cough   2 months
Haemoptysis   2 days

Here the cough has not been complained by the patient, it has been extracted from him. Still then, it should be mentioned in the chief complaints as this will give better information about the illness. This may be a case of pulmonary tuberculosis or a case of bronchogenic carcinoma.

Similarly, for example, a patient comes with the chief complaints of loss of consciousness (say for 2 days), on enquiry it was found that he was also having fever (say for 7 days). Here again even if the chief complaint for the patient is unconsciousness, but for the doctor the chief complaints will be:

Fever   7 days
Loss of consciousness   2 days

This will help in the diagnosis (might be a case of cerebral malaria or meningitis and minimizes the possibility of being other cause of unconsciousness).

Another example will help to understand the issue. A case comes with the complaint of haematemesis (say for 1 day), but on further asking it was revealed that he was having fever with joint pain (say for 5 days). Here his illness started with fever and joint pain. To get relief from pain he took some analgesic which caused erosive gastritis, leading to haematemesis. Haematemesis is not a part of the original illness. It is a complication of the treatment. While treating such a case both aspects have to be considered.

So the true chief complaints will be:

Fever	5 days
Joint pain	5 days
Haematemesis	1 day

Sometimes it becomes difficult to decide from where to start the present illness if it is there since long. If the disease is not diagnosed earlier and he is not on treatment, the total illness should be expressed as one. For example:

A case comes with the complaint of dyspnoea at rest for 5 days, palpitation for 5 days, but on enquiry it was revealed that he is having dyspnoea for 5 years. The better way to express these complaints will be:

Dyspnoea on exertion	5 years
Dyspnoea at rest	5 days
Palpitation	5 days

This will mean that the same disease process has progressed; possibly he has developed arrhythmia (palpitation) which has precipitated congestive heart failure (so dyspnoea at rest).

The same thing can also be expressed while elaborating the history of present illness. For instance:

An established case of diabetes mellitus for so many years comes with complaints of:

Tingling and numbness of both lower limbs 6 months

Tingling and numbness of both upper limbs 1 month

This will mean that the same disease process has progressed (a case of diabetes mellitus has now developed peripheral neuropathy). That he is a case of diabetes mellitus of so many years duration on XYZ treatment or no treatment can be told at the beginning of history of present illness.

On the other hand, if the existing illness does not appear to have any relationship to the present illness, then the long standing illness can be mentioned in the history of past illness. For example:

A case of rheumatic heart disease comes with complains of yellow colouration of conjunctiva, yellow colouration of urine and loss of appetite for one week duration. Here, the patient is suffering possibly from viral hepatitis which has no relationship to his heart ailment. So the heart ailment should be mentioned in the past illness. Similarly, suppose a diagnosed case of bronchial asthma comes with hemiplegia of two days duration, then the bronchial asthma can be included in past illness.

At times the patient tells a lot of complaints in the chief complaints, all need not be significant. If felt minor and insignificant they should be excluded from the chief complaints, however, can be mentioned in the history of present illness.

In evaluating the history of present illness there are some clue points which need elaboration, because they help in diagnosis. These are as follows.

The Starting Complaint

Always emphasis should be given to collect the correct starting complaint. What was the complaint when the patient first felt that he is not well? With the progress of the illness more and more symptoms (even more ominous symptoms) might have been added to the starting complaint. Let us discuss a few examples.

An unconscious patient had fever and neck rigidity. It could be a case of meningitis or a case of subarachnoid haemorrhage. Here what will decide is the starting complaint. If the starting complaint is severe headache (no fever at that time), it is likely to be a case of subarachnoid haemorrhage. Whereas, if the starting complaint is fever; it is likely to be a case of meningitis.

A woman in advanced pregnancy comes with convulsion and loss of consciousness and on examination she was found to have fever also. It could be eclampsia or it could be a case of infective condition of the central nervous system (like encephalitis). If the relatives categorically deny that there was no fever at the beginning of the illness and it all started with convulsion, very likely it is a case of eclampsia of pregnancy (it is to be noted that in a patient with repeated convulsions high blood pressure may not help to diagnose eclampsia, similarly following several episodes of convulsion body temperature may rise even without infection). On the other hand, if the patient was having fever for some days before the onset of convulsion, it is likely to be a case of infection of the central nervous system, like encephalitis. There are many such examples where the starting complaint becomes decisive.

Duration of the Complaints

Often it becomes difficult on the part of the students to clearly determine the duration of the illness. However, a general idea can be made about it from the complaints. For example, if a patient says the duration of illness in terms of months or years, then the onset of the disease is gradual. A patient complains of abdominal pain for 10-12 months (the range he tells is 2 months). Similarly, if a patient complains of dyspnoea for 5 to 6 years (the range itself is one year). This type of presentation suggests chronic nature of the problem and gradual onset of the illness. On the other hand, the patient may be able to tell the exact time and/or date of the onset of the symptoms. Here the nature of the illness is likely to be an acute one. For instance, a patient may say that he felt chest pain on 1st January at 9 am or may say he developed weakness of one half of the body at 5 am on 1st March.

There are certain illnesses which are by nature episodic, like epilepsy, bronchial asthma, episodes of congestive heart failure on existing RHD (Rheumatic Heart Disease), episodes of acute exacerbations of chronic bronchitis, etc. To give best information in these situations it will be better to express as follows:

(a) Bronchial asthma:

Episodic wheezing	10 years
Severe breathlessness	2 days

(b) RHD:

Dyspnoea on exertion	5 years
Dyspnoea at rest	5 days

and so on.

In case of chronic illnesses it may be difficult to decide the exact duration of the illness. Often they get used to live with the problem. They only seek medical attention when the same symptom becomes severe enough to impair their way of living or new symptoms get added to it, so that they cannot do their work. Here they say that the disease has started from the time of their incapacitation. But truly the disease might have started much earlier. On tactful asking the true duration of the illness can be ascertained. Some examples will clarify the issue.

Example 1

A 19-year-old girl comes with the complaint of breathlessness for one month. On examination she was found to be suffering from mitral stenosis. Does it mean that the mitral stenosis has developed within one month? Obviously not. The duration of the illness were revealed in the following way.
Question (Q) by examiner: What are you doing now?
Answer (A) by the patient: Household work.

Q. Why are you not studying?
A. Because of poverty.

Q. From where do you get your drinking water?
A. From the well.

Q. Where is it?
A. It is about half kilometer from my house.

Q. Who brings water for your family?
A. Myself.

Q. What is the size of the pot you are using?
A. About 15 liters capacity.

Q. Are you using the same size pot all the time?
A. Yes.

Q. Are you able to bring the water filled pot to your house at one stretch?

A. No, I have to take rest once or twice on the way.

Q. Why?

A. Because I feel breathless.

Q. How long are you feeling like this?

A. For last one year.

Here even if the girl is complaining of dyspnoea for one month, truly she is having it for last one year.

Example 2

A 34-year-old clerk complains of dyspnoea for one month, so that he is not able to go to work. On examination he was found to have mitral stenosis. Again, does it mean that he is suffering from mitral stenosis for one month? Again; not likely. The true duration of the illness was revealed in the following way.

Q. How far is your office from your house?

A. 2 kilometers.

Q. How do you go to the office?

A. By scooter.

Q. How many storeyed building is your office?

A. Four storeyed.

Q. Is there a lift?

A. No.

Q. In which floor are you working?

A. In ground floor.

Q. How long are you working in the ground floor?
A. For last two years.

Q. Who brought you to the ground floor?
A. I myself have come by applying to the authority.

Q. Why?
A. Because I could not climb stairs to go to the third floor where I was working earlier.

Q. Why?
A. I felt dyspnoeic.

So here again the patient says his illness to be of one month duration though he has got the problem for two years. When he was incapacitated by the symptom, he consulted the doctor. Before that he just modified his lifestyle and went on working, never felt that he has got some physical problem to seek medical help.

These are just two examples. Every day we encounter cases giving ambiguous history, particularly in relation to the duration of the illness. The true duration can be known by analyzing their exact nature of the work and how it has been affected by the illness and how long.

Ascertaining the Genuine Nature of the Complaint

Patient is not a technical man. So he does not understand the implication of what he says. At times it becomes difficult to make out the complaints of the patient. These mis-understandings can lead to erroneous diagnosis. So always try to verify whether the complaint is genuine or not. Students particularly commit this mistake and say that the patient told like this or that. Some complaints are often wrongly interpreted like transient loss of consciousness and convulsions. Let us try to explain how to ascertain the genuine nature of the complaint with some examples.

Convulsions

People often confuse restlessness and abnormal limb movements as convulsion. Ask exactly what happened from the eyewitness. You can show yourself the convulsive movements before the attendants and compare that with what they have seen. Ask whether it occurred while under attention or not. Whether the patient had a fall or not? If there was a fall whether it was associated with injuries or not? If a patient falls knowingly he will try not to hurt himself, at least he will protect the head. He will try to fall by putting his hands on the ground or putting his hip on the ground. If you get a chance to see the fall or the involuntary movements (which the attendants tell to be convulsion), it will be very clear. Other associated features like tongue bite, involuntary passage of urine, twisting of the head, rolling of the eye ball will go in favour of a true convulsion. Fall from sitting or sleeping posture is possible with true and hysterical convulsion; whereas fall from standing posture is more likely to be organic. If at all a person tries to fall from standing posture he will sit first then he will fall. If the fall occurred in a public place (like on the road), it is more likely to be genuine fall. If it occurred in the domestic environment in the presence of others, it may or may not be a genuine fall. In true convulsion, there is a definite pattern of movement of the limbs or body; whereas in hysterical convulsion the movements are often bizarre.

Loss of consciousness: Many of the points discussed under the previous heading will also help in this situation. Often people say that the patient is losing consciousness off and on (several times within a short period), this is not acceptable. This can only be possible in hysterical condition. Sometimes people say that the patient regains consciousness on closure of the nose (this method is to be discouraged). This is not possible in true unconsciousness.

Breathlessness

If a man doing physical labour complains of breathlessness, its genuine nature can be verified by asking how much it affects his work. It may be so that he is no more able to go to work, then the complaint is genuine; because, unless they go to work they may not be able to arrange their daily food. In fact, these people continue to work in the early stages of the disease. At times they change the type of work. I remember a case who was doing physical labour, changed to become a salesman in a small shop. He earned less by changing the work. On asking why he did this; he answered he could not do his earlier work because of dyspnoea.

In a child this can be ascertained how it affects his playing. If he is going to school, ask what game he plays and how efficiently. Is he forced to take rest in the middle or at half time? If he is not a schoolgoing child, ask whether he is able to play satisfactorily with his siblings or children in the neighbourhood. At times the mother may say that the younger child is able to do more work than the elder one; signifying that the complaint of breathlessness of the elder child is genuine.

Weight loss

Often people exaggerate the complaint of weight loss. It is not uncommon to hear the complaint of fifty percent weight loss; which may mean if a person was 50 kg weight earlier now he has become 25 kg. This is not always acceptable or believable. To know whether there is true weight loss or not ask the patient, what was his previous weight and when it was recorded and why it was recorded? From the present weight you can calculate the weight loss over that period. If the patient is not able to tell the previous weight, weight loss can only be assumed. This can also be assessed fairly well from the clothing. If the trouser which has been stitched recently has become too loose so that he has to use belt; or if the number of holes in the belt has been increased recently, then the weight loss is likely to be significant. Similarly, in females looseness of the blouse can be utilized to assess the reliability of weight loss. *Once significant weight loss is established, very likely there is a genuine illness.*

Appetite

Frequently patients complain of loss of appetite. How genuine it is, can be known from the person who ordinarily serves food to him; may be mother or wife or the cook. What is his usual food habit (quantity and quality) and whether there has been any change or not in this habit can be ascertained from them. A person complaining of anorexia for several days but without its affect on the general health of the individual may not be genuine. If anorexia is of short duration, this may not be true, rather there may be associated symptoms of nausea and vomiting as in acute viral hepatitis.

Vomiting

If a patient complains of vomiting off and on for a prolonged period, it is supposed to affect his nutrition and hydration status. If no such effect is noticed, then the complaint is unacceptable; so try to find out some other complaint which is misunderstood as vomiting or it is fictitious vomiting. Each time he might be bringing out little amount of saliva only or there might be retching only. This can be further ensured by asking the patient to collect all the vomitus and produce before you.

Fever and Chill

In relation to fever, confusion arises on the degree of fever and the type of fever (like continued, intermittent or others). Often people say that the patient had very high fever so much so that it was not possible to put the hands on the patient's body. This may or may not be true, because often people exaggerate to emphasize the complaint. If the patient or any other medical personnel has recorded the temperature and it shows that it was really high, then it is alright; if such a record is not available, then no conclusion can be made. Similarly often people say that the type of fever is intermittent. This may be either truly intermittent or falsely intermittent. If the fever subsides under the influence of antipyretics, it is likely to be falsely intermittent. If fever subsides automatically, it is truly intermittent. Each has got its own significance.

In a case of pneumonia a single shaking chill at the beginning is expected. Under such setting if there are repeated chill, it will suggest the development of empyema or lung abscess. But before coming to this conclusion one should see that it is not due to the administration of antipyretics. Because, each time the patient takes antipyretic, fever goes down and as the body regains temperature there occurs chill.

At times people (particularly young females) complain of fever for several days without any other symptoms or any adverse effect on the body, so that they look completely healthy. Before subjecting these cases for detail investigations ask them to maintain a temperature chart at least four to six times a day for a period of at least one week. If the record shows fever, then proceed for investigation. If fever is not recorded, very likely it is psychogenic in nature. I have seen few such cases where by simply asking to record the temperature chart has cured the illness. **Remember that if there is recorded fever in any case, there is organic illness.** Sometimes patients feel sense of warmth (feverishness) in the body without recorded fever. This is possible in certain situations like thyrotoxicosis or in post-menopausal syndrome or intake of certain drugs like nifedipine. At times such feeling is also noticed in malaria and tuberculosis, particularly if it occurs at specified time of the day.

Haemoptysis and Haematemesis
The usual confusion between haematemesis and haemoptysis is always there. Because, whatever blood comes from mouth is considered to be blood vomiting by common people (they do not know the anatomy). So it becomes imperative on the part of the doctor to enquire in detail and decide which is true. The associated symptoms like cough, nausea, the act of vomiting, melaena, encephalopathy, colour of blood,

presence or absence of clot or food material, froth will help to decide. All these points are to be taken into consideration to reach at a conclusion, because one or the other point may not be fulfilled in a particular case. If by chance the patient vomits or spits blood in front of the doctor, then it becomes easier to come to a conclusion.

In relation to the amount of blood loss (whether it is haematemesis or haemoptysis) people often exaggerate. It is not uncommon to hear a complaint that the patient vomited a bucket of blood. But this is not possible; a bucket of blood is not there in human body. So instead of outrightly accepting this, one should verify objectively the amount of blood loss. One should not forget to examine the oral cavity in all such cases. I remember a case who presented with the complaint of haematemesis. But the amount of blood loss he indicated by showing his hand and the absence of melaena, raised doubt about it, she was investigated for haemoptysis yielding no result (X-ray). On re-enquiry he told that he had a convulsion following which he brought out that amount of blood only once. On examination of the oral cavity, there was a tongue bite.

Poisoning
In relation to poisoning also, the relatives often understate the amount of poison ingested. One should never get carried away by these statements. Always assess the amount of poison consumed from the physical signs. However, one must remember some basic things while dealing with a case of poisoning.

- The time gap between the intake and examination.
- Whether he has vomited immediately after intake of the poison or not.
- The time lag between intake of the poison and gastric lavage(if done).
- Has he received any treatment prior to your examination.
- Possibility of cocktail poisoning.

Circumstances under which the Disease Started

In some cases knowing the details of the circumstance under which the illness started will give valuable clue to the diagnosis. A few examples will help to understand this.

A patient of diabetes mellitus on treatment, received the drugs but took less than the amount of food he is supposed to take or vomited immediately after intake of the food and later on was brought in a state of unconsciousness; he is very likely to be suffering from hypoglycemic coma.

A patient who had gone to a malaria endemic area and after few days of returning from there he suffered from fever with altered sensorium, is likely to be suffering from cerebral malaria.

A person went to Delhi during the epidemic of dengue fever and after returning, he suffered from fever with epistaxis, very likely that he has also suffered from dengue.

An elderly person developed chest pain and collapsed while running to catch the train, has most likely suffered from acute myocardial infarction.

A case of subarachnoid haemorrhage was improving well until a day when he went to the toilet and strained for stool and then deteriorated, likely to have had rebleeding.

A school boy brought unconscious without any preceding illness and on enquiry it was found that recently the result of his examination has been declared where he has failed, is likely to have consumed some poison.

I remember a case, (a woman) who suddenly started talking and behaving abnormally from 5 pm of a particular day; before that she was completely alright. That the illness was purely psychogenic was revealed from the history. It was revealed that a previously finalized marriage proposal of her daughter was cancelled by the groom side. This message was received at 5 pm; and since then she started these symptoms.

In a hostel, there were two boys in one room. Both of them used to keep milk in one pot and both of them were drinking from the same pot. One day the first boy drank his part milk and went to play. After some time the second boy came and on going to drink his share of milk found that a house lizard has fallen into it. He did not drink. After two hours the first boy returned and knew from his friend that there was a house lizard in the milk. Since then the first boy started vomiting so much that it required hospitalization. Here the vomiting is psychogenic in origin. Had it been due to some toxic effect, vomiting would have occurred much earlier and the manifestation would not have waited till hearing of the news of falling of the lizard.

A young girl waiting for the bus at the bus stop in the summer season and standing under the sun for a prolonged time fainted suddenly. This is most likely due to vaso vagal syncope.

In a school a teacher felt weakness, anorexia and nausea. On investigation it was found that he was suffering from chronic renal failure. After few months he died. Soon after his death, two of his colleagues came for consultation with exactly similar complaints. Here again the problem is more of psychogenic rather than real (out of fear).

A patient had a fall following which he developed hemiplegia and became unconscious. Here two things are possible. Either the fall is first so that he has developed head injury which has caused hemiplegia or first he developed cerebrovascular accident (causing hemiplegia and unconsciousness) leading to fall. This can be decided taking the circumstances into account which led to fall. Where the person fell down was it slippery? Was it ill lighted? Was it a known or unknown place? Was there any object on which he might have stumbled? Under ordinary circumstances a person with good vision will not fall down on a known path even in darkness unless the path has become slippery or there is something to stumble over.

Associated Complaints

Often the patient comes with more than one complaint. This may be told by the patient frankly or may have to be revealed by tactful questioning. These associated complaints help maximum in reaching at the diagnosis. There are many examples.

Fever
- Associated with cough and expectoration—respiratory infection.

- Associated with jaundice—hepatobiliary disorder, leptospirosis, complicated malaria. It has to be remembered that in viral hepatitis by the time jaundice appears fever subsides.
- Associated with dysuria and frequency—Urinary tract infection.
- Associated with loss of consciousness—CNS infection (cerebral malaria, meningitis, encephalitis, typhoid encephalopathy).

Swelling of the body
- Associated with dyspnoea—congestive heart failure, angioneurotic oedema.
- Associated with jaundice—Subacute hepatic failure, decompensated cirrhosis.
- Associated with oliguria and haematuria—Acute glomerulonephritis.

Breathlessness
- Associated with chest pain—Pneumothorax, pulmonary embolism, acute myocardial infarction.
- Associated with wheezing—Bronchial asthma.
- Associated with cough and sputum production—Chronic bronchitis.
- Associated with haemoptysis—Mitral stenosis, pulmonary infarction.

Joint pain
- Associated with morning stiffness—Rheumatoid arthritis.
- Associated with high fever—Septic arthritis.

- Associated with chronic diarrhea—Inflammatory bowel disease.
  And so on.

Negative History

- Significant negative history should be told in relevant cases. For example:

  In an unconscious patient complete absence of fever practically excludes the possibility of any infective condition. Absence of syncope and angina should be mentioned in all cases of aortic valve disease, as it is required to assess the severity of aortic valve disease. A patient with convulsion, absence of head injury and intoxication should be mentioned. In a patient with ascending paralysis absence of animal bite is required to be mentioned. There are many such examples.

History of Past Illness

> When the clinical observation and the investigation reports go in opposite direction believe the patient (clinical findings).

Past illnesses may have a cause and effect relationship with the present illness or may guide the treatment of the present illness. In this part of the history, history of similar illness and history of significant illnesses should be collected. In every case history of hypertension, diabetes mellitus, tuberculosis and syphilis should be included as these conditions can affect many organs.

There are several illnesses which can occur repeatedly (similar illness). For instance; bronchial asthma, acute exacerbations of chronic bronchitis, bronchiectasis, epileptic attacks, paralytic episodes of multiple sclerosis, migraine, episodes of congestive heart failure, paroxysmal supraventricular tachycardia, haemolytic episodes in congenital haemolytic anaemia; jaundice, fever and abdominal pain of cholangitis and many more.

As it may not be easy to decide which past history will be significant in a particular case, it will be better to ask the patient or his relatives to enumerate all the major illnesses he has suffered from childhood including major accidents and surgeries. From them one has to screen out which is important which is not. Before accepting a diagnosis told by the patient several aspects should be considered. He should be asked to produce the documents related to previous illness. If he is not able to do that, ask about the symptoms with their duration, reports of investigations if he is able to remember or the treatment he received with its duration. This cross verification of past illness is required because often the patients tell the name of the disease or condition, whatever they have remembered or understood which may not be scientifically accurate. For example, if a patient gives history of rheumatic fever, ascertain it by asking at what age it occurred; which joints were affected, how severe was the joint pain, whether there was fleeting character or not, whether penicillin prophylaxis was advised or not. If a diagnosis of nephritis is told, ask whether there was diminished urination or not, whether there was haematuria or not, whether there was swelling of the face and legs or not.

There are several significant past conditions and diseases which has got relationships with the present ailment. With increase in the level of knowledge in medicine one can know what is significant in what conditions. Some examples are given here. In a case of heart disease past history of rheumatic fever, in a case of amoebic liver abscess history of amoebic dysentery, in a case of tubercular meningitis history of tuberculosis (often partially treated), in a case of infective endocarditis recent history of dental procedure, in a case of upper GI bleeding past history of portal hypertension or acid peptic disease, in a case of lung abscess history of unconsciousness or general anaesthesia, in a case of chronic renal failure history of repeated urinary tract infection or obstructive uropathy are significant.

Collecting History of Diabetes Mellitus

From the symptoms like polyuria, polyphagia and polydipsia one can suspect about diabetes mellitus. But these classical features are only found in cases of type I diabetes mellitus. However, majority of the cases being type II diabetes mellitus, these features may not be found. Polyuria is due to glycosuria and polydipsia is due to polyuria (causing volume loss). To have polyuria the blood glucose level has to go above the renal threshold. So if there is hyperglycaemia of more than 180 mg/dl (renal threshold), polyuria and polydipsia can be found irrespective of the type of diabetes mellitus. There are many more symptoms from which diabetes mellitus can be suspected only. Often we see cases who have been diagnosed as diabetes mellitus on the basis of presence of reducing substances in the urine. This is not only incorrect, but also it can be dangerous at times. If a patient gives history of diabetes mellitus, enquire on what basis he has been told to be diabetic. If they produce documentary evidence of diabetes mellitus or if they remember the level of blood glucose (done at a reliable laboratory), it may be accepted. At times the patient shows documentary evidence of hyperglycemia tested at a previous occasion, but a fresh report does not support this; the previous report need not be outrightly rejected. This is possible under certain situations; like honeymoon phase of Type I diabetes, Gestational diabetes, if the patient has developed advanced diabetic nephropathy, drug-induced diabetes, etc.

Collecting History of Tuberculosis

That the patient was suffering from tuberculosis can be known from the previous treatment records, X-rays, sputum examination reports, etc. If such reports are not available, previous history of prolonged fever, persistent cough (more than two/ three weeks), haemoptysis, weight loss, etc. (single or combination) should be enquired. The drugs prescribed may also help to decide whether these were antitubercular drugs. Consumption of combipacks, three /four tablets advised to be taken together in the morning, duration of treatment for six to nine months; orange colour urine after consumption of the drugs; all may help to decide that it was an antitubercular regimen. Remember that people often do not want to reveal that they suffered or are suffering from tuberculosis and invariably they say that they have completed the drug therapy even if they have taken for a few days only.

History of Hypertension

In a country like India history of hypertension is obtained in a confusing manner. Often people (both educated and uneducated) say that they had/have blood pressure (not even high blood pressure); which does not carry any meaning.

At times people say that they are having low blood pressure. The concept of low blood pressure is also very vague. Genuine persistent low blood pressure due to an organic cause is extremely rare. It is also found that people conclude themselves that they are suffering from hypertension from the symptoms like reeling of head without any measurement of blood pressure. If the patients tell like that without mentioning the correct recording, it should not be accepted. It is not uncommon to notice that people do not remember the exact figure of blood pressure and often tell wrongly. Always emphasis should be given to produce the documentary evidence of hypertension. At times people are able to remember the names of the drugs from which it can be presumed whether the patient was hypertensive or not. If a normal recording of blood pressure is found always ascertain whether the patient is on the drugs or off the drugs. For example, BP 130/80 mmHg (with amlodipine 10 mg).

History of Syphilis

Syphilis in earlier days was the single most important disease to involve almost all organs. Primarily it is a sexually transmitted disease. Unless carefully and tactfully asked people do not reveal it. In fact, most people do not tell freely about any sexual problems. This is more so in females. To discuss these matters an environment conducive for such discussion should be made. Following the sexual act whether there was any penile sore or not? Whether the sore was painful or painless? Whether they received any treatment or not? Because, Spirochetes are highly sensitive to many commonly used antibiotics, a course of antibiotic may eradicate the organism. In male the commonest site of primary chancre is over the penis (glans and shaft), so one can see it and take medical help. But in females the common site of primary chancre is over the cervix, which goes un- noticed and remains untreated. So presence or absence of sore in female is less significant.

Though syphilis has lost its significance in the post-antibiotic era, another sexually transmitted disease with multi-organ involvement has emerged. That is AIDS. So the sexual history has not lost its significance even now.

Family History

> The simplest way to improve the power of observation is to note how a person differs from a normal man.

Certain diseases are likely to occur in many members of the family. Presence of similar illness in other members of the family helps in reaching at a diagnosis. These categories of illnesses can be divided into two groups:
a. Genetically transmitted diseases
b. Familial clustering of diseases

Genetically Transmitted Diseases

There are many diseases which are transmitted genetically. A family tree should be drawn to know the pattern of transmission. It is to be kept in mind that a genetically transmitted condition can occur in a person without similar illness in the family due to mutation. While analyzing a genetically transmitted condition one has to keep in mind that a particular condition may not express completely in all cases (full expression or partial expression). If a genetically transmitted condition is suspected history of consanguineous marriage in the family should be enquired. Autosomal recessive disorders are likely to manifest in such situation. A short list of genetically transmitted diseases is given herewith.

Autosomal Dominant Disorders

- Adult polycystic kidney disease
- Huntington's chorea
- Most of the heritable connective tissue disorders like Marfan's syndrome, osteogenesis imperfecta, etc.
- Multiple neurofibromatosis
- Hereditary spherocytosis
- Familial hypercholesterolemia
- Myotonia dystrophica
- Acute intermittent porphyria and so on.

Autosomal Recessive Disorders

- Albinism
- Wilson's disease
- Sickle cell anaemia
- Beta thalassaemia
- Cystic fibrosis
- Friedreich's ataxia
- Haemochromatosis
- Phenylketonuria and homocystinuria and many other inborn errors of metabolism.

X-linked Recessive Disorders

- Haemophilia
- G6PD deficiency

    Ocular albinism
- Colour blindness
- HGPRT deficiency and others.

X-linked Dominant Disorders (Rare)

- Orofaciodigital syndrome
- Focal dermal hypoplasia
- Incontigentia pigmenti
- Hypophosphatemic rickets

Familial Clustering of Diseases

Some diseases occur in many members of the families due to exposure to similar environment. Here genetics do not play a role. Genetically dissimilar people can also suffer from the illness if they stay together. All the members take food from same kitchen, all take water from the same pot, all remain in the similar housing condition and all breathe similar air. So familial clustering of diseases is mostly water borne, food mediated or air borne in nature. Food-mediated diseases may be due to nutritional toxins or germs or nutritional deficiency. Deficiency diseases are more likely to manifest in them who require the nutritional factor more, like children, pregnant women and lactating mothers. Dietary toxins may be two types; acute toxins (for instance, food poisoning) and chronic toxins (for instance, lathyrism). Acute toxin-mediated diseases are more likely to affect all those who have consumed the contaminated food, though the dose of exposure also determines the severity of manifestation. Chronic toxin-mediated diseases are more dependent on the duration of exposure.

As the elder members in a family are likely to be exposed for longer time, these types of diseases are more common in them.

At times many members of an institution can suffer from similar illness due to similar reasons as in case of a family. For example, many members of a hostel may suffer from common water-borne diseases like typhoid fever or infective hepatitis.

Sometimes diseases need not be confined to one family. Many families may get affected from similar illness. This is particularly true for epidemic diseases. Though these epidemic diseases are mostly infective, but may be nutritional in origin like epidemic dropsy. Only one member of a family may suffer from a disease (say- hepatitis), but if the history reveals that few other cases of similar illness have occurred in the near by families, it will suggest an epidemic, may be a mini-epidemic.

6

Personal History

> Never leave a patient receiving
> blood transfusion alone.
> Basically it is a tissue transplant.

Many people have many things personal to them, many ways of living personal to them. These personal things at times contribute to the causation of the diseases and so detection of all these personal things can help in the diagnosis of the ailments. Though there are many personal things, few only contribute to the causation of the disease and these things will be discussed only.

Food Habit

Ask for the type of food one takes, whether he gets two/three full meals per day or not? What are the usual contents of his food? From this one can assess whether one is suffering from malnutrition or not. Remember that malnutrition-related problems rarely occur to a single nutritional factor. People have personal preference and dislike for food. There may be food allergy too. Ask for any particular reason for the dislike for the food. Dislike for a particular food may be due to food allergy or intolerance. People taking excess of coffee may develop reflux oesophagitis. Excess of tea can produce supraventricular ectopics. Those who are strictly vegetarian (vegan) may suffer from vitamin B_{12} deficiency. Frequency and regularity in food intake may be required to be known for prescription of certain drugs. If history of food intolerance (wheat products in cases of gluten enteropathy) or food allergy is found, they should be advised to avoid such food. Before doing this one should be sure that it is true; because people often misunderstand some other problem with that of food-related problem. Similarly if a patient has got an allergic disorder he should be asked to observe if any particular food exacerbates the disorder. Other food-related problems may be due to dietary toxins. So enquire any such food taken for a long time as happens with *Khesari dal* (Lathyrism).

Addiction and Habituation

Ask for any type of addiction or dependence. The commonly encountered such things are alcohol, opium, several drugs, tobacco in various forms and so on.

Alcohol

This is one of the commonest addictions throughout the world. It can cause multiple health problems in addition to social problems. It can affect the GI system (gastritis, pancreatitis, fatty liver, hepatitis, cirrhosis of liver), the nervous system (peripheral neuropathy, Korsakoff's psychosis, Wernicke's encephalopathy, delirium tremens, cerebellar degeneration, dementia and others). Alcoholics are more likely to suffer from aspiration pneumonia. The duration and amount of alcohol consumption should be enquired. Often people say that they have left taking alcohol. But on further enquiry it can be revealed that they might have left for a few days only. In fact, history of leaving and resuming alcohol for several times may be obtained.

Smoking

Ask for the type of smoke one uses (*bidi*, cigarette, *Hucca* etc). More important is the amount and the duration of smoking. Sometimes people smoke keeping the burning end inside the mouth. Enquire about the passive smoking too. Patient might be taking tobacco in other forms also, enquire about it as because tobacco in any form is bad for health. Some of the common non-smoking method of tobacco consumptions are brushing the teeth (*gudakhu*), snuff (*nasa*), betel chewing (*pan*).There are several problems associated with smoking. The respiratory problems like chronic bronchitis, bronchogenic carcinoma, smoker's cough, cardiovascular problems like coronary artery disease (CAD), peripheral vascular disease (Buerger's disease). Smoking is associated with increased incidence of almost all types of malignancies particularly lungs, oropharyngeal and oesophageal.

Opium

Consumption of opium itself may not cause any ailment, but it can mask the manifestations of diseases. These patients are often constipated; their pupil size even in physiological state may be little constricted. They do not respond to ordinary doses of analgesics and sedatives.

Drugs

Various types of drugs can lead to habit formation. The commonly abused drugs are narcotics and benzodiazepines. If the drugs are taken intravenously, it increases the chances of suffering from infective endocarditis (often right sided and may be by uncommon organisms) and glomerulonephritis. In an intoxicated state they are more prone to suffer from aspiration pneumonia and injuries (often head injuries). Because of their bad association they are more likely to suffer from tuberculosis and AIDS.

Sleep

The habit of sleeping varies from person to person. Ask when he goes to sleep and when he gets up? Is the sleep refreshing? Is he habituated to take a nap in the daytime? Is there any recent change in the habit of sleeping? If yes, is there any obvious cause? For example, following birth of a newborn often parents have disturbed sleep. However, one of the commonest causes of insomnia is presence of physical ailments and an unfavourable environment. So always look for any physical illness, particularly a condition which causes orthopnoea or a painful condition. An anxious or mentally disturbed person does not go to sleep easily (induction), gets a light sleep with dreams and often gets up early and fails to go to sleep again. Some people by nature take short sleep, but this may be enough for them provided it keeps them refreshed. Some people go to sleep late and also get up late. Their biological clock gets tuned to this pattern, so it does not affect the body or mind provided the quantity and quality of sleep is normal.

Excessive sleep occurs in hypothalamic disorders, Pickwickian syndrome or under the influence of drugs. Excessive sleep can also be due to sleep deprivation.

Reversal of sleep rhythm (night time insomnia and daytime somnolence) occurs in old age, as an early feature of hepatic encephalopathy and nocturnal sleep loss.

Bowel and Bladder

Bowel and bladder habits often vary from person to person. Some people have the habit of defaecation once only in the morning, some have the habit of going two or three times all in the morning, some people have the habit of going once in the morning and once in the evening. All these are normal. Because the normal bowel habit is so different, enquire about any recent change in the habit. Even recent change in bowel habit may not be significant unless a recent change in dietary habit and consumption of drugs are excluded. Pathological cause of recent change in bowel habit (usually constipation) may be due to colorectal malignancy. Recent onset diarrhoea is often due to infection.

Bladder habit often differs in physiological state due to difference in the intake of water. Women have a tendency to evacuate bladder less frequently than males. Disturbance in bladder habit may take several forms like increased frequency of urination, polyuria, oliguria, hesitancy, urgency, dysuria, incontinence, retention, etc.

Socioeconomic Status

The influence of socioeconomic status on the causation of diseases is indirect. Poor socioeconomic status leads to poor housing condition, poor diet and poor hygiene. Hence, various infections and infestations and nutritional deficiency conditions are more frequently encountered in them. High socio-economic status leads to sedentary lifestyle, intake of food rich in fat; both causing obesity and the related problems.

Socioeconomic status is also important for planning the investigations and treatment. Always attempts should be made to limit the total expenditure in every case, particularly in a poor man. For example, a poor man suffers from acute myeloid leukaemia (AML) and comes for treatment. If scientifically he is planned for treatment, the cost of treatment will be so high that he may have to sell all his property for few courses of chemotherapy only and ultimately he will die. After his death his family members will be left to begging. Such cases should be discouraged for any treatment. They should be explained the net consequences of the disease and its therapy. Under such situation the decision of not treating the patient is wiser than to treat him. I want to quote one statement in this regard. Hutchison himself wrote: "From *making the cure of the disease more grievous than the endurance thereof, good lord deliver us." Under no circumstance the treatment of an ailment should be more cumbersome and painful than the disease itself.*

Socioeconomic status should be assessed from the total income of a family and its expenditure. If there is only one earning member in a family and there are many dependent members to be taken care of, the socioeconomic status may not be good. On the other hand, if all the members are earning (even if less), then their socioeconomic status may be fairly good. Assessing the economic status of salaried people is not difficult. In farmers economic status should be assessed from how many acres of landed property they have got and how many crops they grow and what is the annual yield. In case of daily labourers things are very obvious. While evaluating the social status one should try to know about the house (type of house, type of ventilation, lighting), and about the usual sources of drinking water. Poor housing condition may be contributing to repeated upper and lower respiratory tract infections, attacks of bronchial asthma and so on. Unsafe drinking water may cause several water-borne diseases.

Marital Status

It is required to know about the marital status of the person for several reasons. Though marriage itself has nothing directly to do with any disease, but matrimonial disharmony is a common cause of psychiatric illness. Physical illness in a spouse may be a cause of the matrimonial disharmony (often the illness may be trivial). Often one spouse may become afraid at the illness of the other spouse. Here they should be clearly explained the nature of the illness and the modalities of treatment. Even they can be advised how to adjust with each other in day-to-day life. If one partner becomes Hepatitis B positive, the other partner should be immediately vaccinated.

If somebody becomes father at an advanced age, the child may develop Marfan's syndrome and if somebody becomes mother at an advanced age, the child may suffer from Down's syndrome. Because diabetics can develop impotence later on in the course of the illness, they are to be advised to complete the family earlier. There are some conditions like Eisenmenger's syndrome, Tetralogy of Fallot, Co-arctation of the aorta, Primary pulmonary hypertension, where the women are advised to avoid pregnancy; because these women do not tolerate pregnancy and delivery well. If there is a chronic illness in the parents (not necessarily genetically transmitted disease), often they ask if the illness is likely to occur in their children. Things should be clearly revealed and explained to them. If it is a genetically transmitted condition, it should also be told what the probability of the offspring developing the disease is and how it can be detected before birth if possible.

In all married individuals enquire about the number of children and their health. Infertile couples often come with various psychosomatic illnesses.

Exercise

Ask if the patient does some physical exercise (includes physical work) or not. Note how he is tolerating the exercise. Whether he has stopped or modified the exercise; if so is there any specific reason. If he is habituated to do some physical exercise, it is required to instruct him (even if not asked) if he can do the same after some major illnesses particularly cardiovascular and respiratory illnesses; if so what is the ideal time? Patients of coronary artery disease and subarachnoid haemorrhage should avoid isometric exercise.

Pets

Many people keep various types of pets. If the patient keeps one enquire about it. Whether proper care is taken or not? Whether properly vaccinated or not? Bird droppings can precipitate asthmatic attack, bird handlers can suffer from ornithosis. Keeping unvaccinated dogs or cats may lead to bites or scratches which can lead to rabies, unhealthy dogs can transmit hydatid disease.

Menstrual and Obstetrics History

> The absolute sciences in Medicine are Anatomy,
> Physiology and Biochemistry. Learn clinical
> medicine keeping them in the background.

In every female in the childbearing age group menstrual history and obstetrics history must be taken irrespective of the type of illness (medical, surgical or gynaecological). The age of menarche and menopause should be ascertained. Usually menarche occurs between the ages of 12 and 13 years. If it does not occur by 20 years of age, it should be called delayed menarche, which may be due to various local and systemic diseases. Menarche before the age of 8 years is called precocious puberty which may be due to certain brain tumors, hormone-secreting ovarian tumors, hypothyroidism, post-meningitic and encephalitic state. Similarly menopause commonly occurs between 45 and 55 years (mean age 47 years). When it occurs before 40 years, it is called premature menopause. Delayed menopause may be due to conditions like endometrial carcinoma and uterine fibroid.

Normal menstrual cycle has got two parts; the cycles and the flow period. The length of the cycle varies from 25 to 30 days with a mean of 28 days. The average duration of flow varies from 3 to 5 days and the amount is between 50 ml and 200 ml. Normal menstrual blood does not clot. Passage of clots usually signifies excess flow. Flow more than 8 days also indicates excess flow (menorrhagia). Menorrhagia ordinarily suggests local disease in the uterus like fibroid, genital tuberculosis, endometriosis, adenomyosis, etc. but can be due to systemic illnesses like bleeding disorders, hypothyroid state and so on. Scanty menstruation is also a common complaint. Here the duration of menstrual flow is one or two days only. If the cycles are regular, this alone does not cause any problem, hence needs only reassurance. However, if it is associated with irregular/ infrequent menstrual cycles, ovarian failure/ subfunction should be thought of. A normal menstrual cycle almost suggests a normal pituitary, ovarian and uterine axis. Disorder in the cycle signifies defect in the pituitary ovarian axis.

Some of the common disorders of cycle are polymenor- rhoea and metrorrhagia. In polymenorrhoea the length of the cycle is shortened to two to three weeks. It may be associated with excess bleeding during the flow; when it is called polymenorrhagia. These types of problems are encoun- tered at menarche, menopause and a few cycles following delivery. Metrorrhagia means there is irregular acyclical bleeding; there is bleeding in between the normal cycles. Mostly this type of abnormality is found in genital malignancies (uterine/ cervical/ vaginal); but may be due to submucous fibroid, uterine polyp and cervical polyp.

The commonest cause of amenorrhoea in childbearing age group is pregnancy. So in amenorrhoea in this age group pregnancy must be excluded irrespective of the marital status. In fact, family members do not accept pregnancy in an unmarried girl or widows. This has put the doctors in awkward position several times and often diagnosis has been delayed. Besides pregnancy there are several systemic diseases which can lead to amenorrhoea like thyrotoxicosis, advanced genital tuberculosis, Sheehan's syndrome, consumption of oral contraceptive pills, prolonged intake of tranquilizers, Addison's disease, adrenal tumors, long-standing diabetes mellitus, anaemia, chronic renal diseases and so on.

Women very often do not speak out freely about their genital problems. So it is better to ask directly certain questions particularly genital discharge (other than menstrual flow). This often helps to pick up cases of carcinoma cervix early.

Pregnancy must be excluded in every female cases of reproductive age group because investigations (particularly radiological) should be done judiciously. Prescribing for pregnant woman needs special precaution. These restrictions are more important if it is early pregnancy. Some general guidelines of prescribing in pregnancy are:

- Avoid all drugs as far as possible
- Prescribe those drugs which have been declared to be safe
- The dose and duration should not exceed that is compatible with achieving the therapeutic goal
- If decided to prescribe a drug which has not declared to be safe, the patient and the guardians should be informed and explained the necessity of such prescription.

- If the drug or the procedure is likely to be too hazardous, termination of pregnancy can be advised.

It may so happen that a woman has conceived in the continuing cycle so that there is no history of amenorrhoea. For example, last menstrual period (LMP) was on 1st April. She comes for consultation for some illness on 25th April. There is no amenorrhoea yet. But ovulation has supposed to occur around 14th of the same month (thinking it to be a 28 days' cycle) and if she has conceived around that time she might be carrying a pregnancy of 8-10 days' duration. Exposing her to radiation or to potentially harmful drugs during this highly vulnerable period should be avoided. To avoid such cases the rule of ten days should be obeyed. The first ten days from the day of menstruation are the safest period for any investigation or for any treatment. Grossly, it can be told that the first half of the cycle is safe and the second half is unsafe.

Menstrual history is not only important for medical illnesses but also needed for surgical conditions. For instance, a rupture ectopic pregnancy or a red degeneration of the fibroid can be confused with other acute abdominal conditions.

Obstetrics history is equally important to assess the severity of a long-standing illness; often may help to decide the exact duration of the illness (how the previous pregnancies have been tolerated). Repeated stillbirth and abortion may be due to some underlying illnesses. Whether the present pregnancy is valuable or not can be known from the obstetrics history and accordingly treatment can be planned. Other medical illnesses related to childbirth are cortical venous sinus thrombosis, peripartum cardiomyopathy, etc.

8

Treatment History

> A patient developing a new complaint while on treatment, attribute it to the drugs rather than to the disease.

History of medical and surgical treatment should be obtained from all patients. When ever possible ask to produce the records of previous treatments and operations. Previous treatments might be having direct bearing with the present illness. For example, if a case has received Chloromycetin earlier and now comes with hypoplastic anaemia, it may be causally related. If a patient had gastrectomy earlier and now comes with anaemia, he might have developed megaloblastic anaemia due to deficiency of vitamin B_{12}. There are many such examples. Even treatment has got direct effect on the present illness. The signs and symptoms of the present illness may get modified because of treatment. If a case has received antipyretics recently, he may not have fever at the time of examination, if a case of diabetes mellitus is on antidiabetic drugs, he may not have symptoms of diabetes, even his blood sugar assessment may be normal (but does not exclude diabetes); if a case of hypertension is on antihypertensive drugs, his present blood pressure measurement may be normal (does not exclude hypertension). If a case is getting beta-blocker his resting heart rate may be slower, if a case is getting parasympatholytic drugs his pupil may be little dilated. So if you are examining a case who is receiving some form of medication, always due consideration should be given to their effect on the existing disease process.

Similarly, if a patient is on treatment with certain drugs, before declaring that the drug is not effective one should be sure that the drug has been taken in adequate dose and for adequate duration. On the contrary, if the drug has been taken adequately (dose and duration) and the patient has not shown satisfactory response, there is no meaning of continuing the same drugs (rather change the drug or add some other drug). At times continuation of certain drugs without knowing how long he is continuing the drugs may lead to toxic effects, particularly the drugs which have low therapeutic window (digoxin, anticoagulants). There are some drugs which are to be continued for a long time like antiasthmatic drugs, drugs for heart failure, antiepileptic drugs, antianginal drugs and others. Abrupt withdrawal of these drugs may lead to exacerbation of the underlying illness, at times may result in fatal outcome. Abrupt withdrawal of glucocorticosteroids after a prolonged course may cause acute adrenal failure. Abrupt withdrawal of beta-blocker in a patient of coronary heart disease may precipitate acute myocardial infarction.

While taking the treatment history do not rely on the name of the drugs told by the patients, because they do not tell correctly. So always try to see the prescription and try to physically verify the drugs if he is having with him. Even if the drugs have been prescribed and dispensed correctly, often patients take them in a confusing manner (particularly illiterate people). This happens mostly if there are many medicines in the prescription. At times patients themselves modify the dose giving various explanations. All these aspects are to be looked for in the evaluation of the treatment history.

If a patient develops an adverse drug reaction to any particular drug (for example, anaphylaxis or exfoliative dermatitis); a written warning card (if possible laminated) should be issued to him with the instruction to carry it with him all the time and to produce it before any doctor for any consultation.

In case of infants it may be required to know the medications the mother received during pregnancy and lactation.

All doctors are supposed to give the details of the treatment at the time of discharge or referral. Even presumptive treatment, therapeutic trial, etc. should be mentioned to avoid confusion later on. These things are very important in referral hospitals because rarely they get virgin cases.

Often students do the mistake of seeing the referral slip first before they themselves see the case. This is likely to misguide them towards jumping at a conclusion which may be wrong. This practice blunts the development of their own thought and judgment process. Rather they should take thorough history and do detail examination, come to a conclusion and later on they can verify with the treatment papers or referral slip as the case may be.

9

History in Cardiovascular Disorders

> In relation to treating diarrhoea with dehydration, the basic difference between a general doctor and a specialist doctor is, the latter knows when to stop the IV fluid.

The components of a cardiovascular diagnosis are:

- Aetiological
- Anatomical (structural)
- Haemodynamic effects (like pulmonary arterial hypertension, congestive cardiac failure)
- Specific complications (like infective endocarditis, arrhythmia)
- Functional status (expressed as NYHA class)

Many of these aspects can be known from a carefully taken history. In the history following points as described below are to be collected.

HISTORY OF PRESENT ILLNESS

From history one can suspect that the case might be having a cardiovascular problem if he comes with any of the following chief complaints as single or in combination.

- Dyspnoea
- Swelling of the body
- Chest pain
- Syncope
- Palpitation
- Haemoptysis
- Fever
- Neurological deficit
- Repeated respiratory infection

Of these the first six are most important.

Dyspnoea

People express dyspnoea by several words like breathlessness, shortness of breath, not getting enough air, etc. In addition to diseases of the cardiovascular system (CVS) dyspnoea may be due to respiratory cause or may be due to anaemia also. Though all dyspnoea increases on exertion, but this is more often seen in cardiovascular condition. In CVS dyspnoea indicates the disease is in the left side of the heart (aorta, aortic valve, left ventricle, mitral valve and rarely left atrium). The basic mechanism is elevated left atrial pressure which is reflected into the pulmonary venous system leading to pulmonary venous congestion (hypertension). Dyspnoea is not a symptom of the disease in the right side of the heart, where pulmonary circulation is underloaded. In fact, the severity of dyspnoea decreases with the onset of right-sided heart failure. Severity of dyspnoea should be categorized into NYHA class. The mildest one is Class I and the most severe one is the Class IV. If the dyspnoea is solely dependent on the severity of the underlying heart disease, it will gradually progress from Class I to Class IV). But at times we encounter cases where the severity of dyspnoea jumps one or two steps. For example, a case can go from Class I to Class IV bypassing II and III. Whenever such a history is obtained one should try to find out a precipitating cause (onset of arrhythmia, infective endocarditis, fresh attack of rheumatic carditis, withdrawal of anti-failure drugs, systemic infection particularly respiratory infection, etc). Once the precipitating factor is controlled the patient will go back to the original NYHA Class.

Variants of dyspnoea are paroxysmal nocturnal dyspnoea (PND) and orthopnoea. PND typically occurs two to three hours after actual sleep. If the patient goes into actual sleep for about three hours even in daytime, he can develop PND; whereas if he does not go to actual sleep even in night time, he may not develop PND. Hence, the nocturnal is truly misnomer. PND is nothing but a miniature pulmonary oedema, indicates more severe pulmonary venous hypertension.

As the disease (left-sided heart disease, hence the pulmonary venous pressure) progresses further, patient becomes dyspnoeic in lying down position and feels better in upright posture like sitting. This is called orthopnoea. Often the patient gives the history that he passes the whole night reclining on something (several pillows, wall, etc). He may prefer to sit near the edge of the cot with legs hanging down.

Chest Pain

Chest pain is a common cardiovascular complaint. Chest pain due to heart conditions are mainly due to coronary artery disease (CAD), pericarditis or dissecting aneurysm of aorta.

The pain of CAD is known as angina pectoris which has got specific features. It is primarily retrosternal in site. The character of pain is not properly described by most people. Various types of words are used by various people. Oppressive feelings, sense of suffocation, sense of heaviness, sense of squeezing and so on are the commonly used words. Often an emotional aspect of the feeling can be observed in the facial expression of the patient. In fact, the patient may start weeping while describing the pain and he may say that he had a feeling of the end of life. While describing he may make a fist and move over the sternum. This not only suggests that the pain is retrosternal in location, but also it is squeezing in type. In stable angina patient will be forced to take rest, but in acute myocardial infarction and unstable angina patient may become restless in a vague attempt to get relief (stable angina, unstable angina and myocardial infarction are the spectrum of the clinical manifestations of CAD). Duration of the anginal pain is usually a few minutes. But in unstable angina and myocardial infarction pain may persist for several minutes. Anginal pain radiates to left shoulder, left upper limb along the ulnar border, can radiate to the right shoulder and arm, can radiate to the neck up to the mandible, can radiate down to the epigastric area. Conventionally, it is told that anginal pain does not go above the lower jaw and does not go below the umbilicus. Anginal pain starts or aggravates on exertion or emotion and is relieved by taking rest and nitrates. Pain of oesophageal spasm can be relieved by nitrate, but it has no relation to exertion or emotion and is not necessarily relieved by rest. Pain of myocardial infarction and unstable angina may start at rest and may not be relieved by nitrates always. Associated symptoms like profuse sweating, desire to defaecate, breathlessness, syncope suggest occurrence of myocardial infarction. Typical pain of CAD may not always be felt. It may be felt as dyspnoea, fatigability or palpitation; all are known as angina equivalent.

Pain of pericarditis is more or less identical to angina in relation to location and radiation, but it is more persistent, not associated with other symptoms, not relieved by rest or nitrates. It can be relieved by sitting up and leaning forward, can be aggravated by deglutition.

Pain of dissecting aneurysm of aorta is severe enough to mimic myocardial infarction. Sweating and other associated symptoms of myocardial infarction may occur. The difference is this pain is tearing in character and it radiates to the back between the two scapulae.

Swelling of the Body

Patients of heart disease may come with complaint of swelling of the body. This may be due to right-sided heart failure, pericardial effusion, constrictive pericarditis, restrictive cardio-myopathy, tricuspid valve diseases like tricuspid stenosis and tricuspid regurgitation. In all these conditions the primary factor giving rise to oedema formation is the increased hydrostatic pressure. So the swelling appears first in the dependent parts; legs if the patient is ambulatory, back of the thighs or over the sacrum if the patient is lying down. If dyspnoea preceded the swelling of the body, it is likely to be due to heart failure. Disproportionate accumulation of fluid in the peritoneum (ascites) suggests a condition like tricuspid stenosis or regurgitation, constrictive pericarditis and restrictive cardiomyopathy. In all these conditions jugular veins are engorged (also see GI and urinary system).

Syncope

Syncope is transient loss of consciousness due to sudden decrease in the cerebral blood flow. The commonest cause of syncope is vasovagal syncope. Of the organic causes of syncope cardiovascular cause comes first. Left ventricular outflow tract (LVOT) obstruction like aortic stenosis and hypertrophic obstructive cardiomyopathy (HOCM) are the common causes of cardiac syncope. Presence of syncope in these conditions suggests advanced stage of the disease. Syncope can occur due to cardiac arrhythmias, particularly ventricular tachyarrhythmias as seen in long QT syndrome (Torsades de pointes) and due to marked bradycardia as occurs in complete heart block and sick sinus syndrome. A syncopal attack in the setting of bradycardia is known as Stokes-Adams attacks (SA attacks). The basic difference between syncope and SA attacks is that syncope does not occur in lying down posture (always occurs in upright posture);

whereas SA attacks can occur in any posture. In fact, syncope in LVOT obstruction occurs on exertion (effort syncope). LVOT obstruction as well as arrhythmia can cause syncope in cases of HOCM.

Other less common cardiac causes of syncope are acute myocardial infarction, Tetralogy of Fallot (TOF), ball valve thrombus in mitral stenosis. In acute myocardial infarction syncope may be due to sudden fall in the blood pressure or due to arrhythmia.

Palpitation

Palpitation is the feeling of own heart beat. Palpitation may be due to tachycardia of any cause, due to arrhythmia (usually at the time of change in rhythm) or due to large stroke volume states like aortic regurgitation, mitral regurgitation, ventricular septal defect, etc. If it is due to large stroke volume state it will be persistent (though it can be more marked in left lateral position). If the palpitation is paroxysmal, it is likely to be due to arrhythmia or tachycardia (as in paroxysmal supraventricular tachycardia (PSVT) and pheochromocytoma).

Haemoptysis

Haemoptysis is commonly due to respiratory diseases, but it can be due to certain cardiovascular illnesses. Mitral stenosis is by far the commonest cardiovascular cause. Haemoptysis is seen in the early stage of mitral stenosis. Frequency of haemoptysis decreases after the development of pulmonary arterial hypertension. Other situations where haemoptysis occurs are primary pulmonary hypertension (PPH),

Eisenmenger's syndrome, TOF. A cardiovascular case remaining bedridden for a long time can develop pulmonary embolism and haemoptysis.

Fever

Fever is an uncommon cardiovascular complaint. It can occur in infective endocarditis, fresh attack of rheumatic process, left atrial myxoma, acute pericarditis, pyopericardium. Low-grade fever can occur in myocardial infarction. Because cardiac conditions are infrequent causes of fever, they often present as pyrexia of unknown origin (PUO).

Neurological Deficit

Neurological deficit in cardiovascular illnesses are mostly due to cerebral embolism. Type of neurological deficit depends on the site of lodgment of the embolus. Mitral stenosis, cardiomyopathy, mural thrombus in myocardial infarction, vegetation embolism in infective endocarditis, tumor cell embolism in left atrial myxoma, paradoxical embolism in conditions with right to left shunt (TOF) are the causes which predispose to embolism. In all these conditions the neurological deficit is abrupt in onset. Focal neurological deficit with convulsion can occur in children with cyanotic congenital heart diseases due to development of brain abscess.

Respiratory Infections

Repeated lower respiratory tract infection occurs in children with left to right shunt like ventricular septal defect (VSD), atrial septal defect (ASD) and patent ductus arteriosus (PDA).

So-called winter bronchitis can occur several times in cases of mitral stenosis. In all these conditions the respiratory infection may take the form of bronchitis, broncopneumonia or frank pneumonia.

Cyanosis

Cyanosis is an uncommon mode of presentation of cardiovascular illnesses. It is usually noticed by the physicians when the patient is brought for some other problem. Often it is associated with thickening of the finger tips (clubbing). In cardiovascular illnesses there can be central as well as peripheral cyanosis. Peripheral cyanosis is associated with congestive heart failure. Central cyanosis (where both warm parts as well as exposed parts are affected) is seen in cases of cyanotic congenital heart diseases like TOF, pulmonary atresia, tricuspid atresia, double outlet right ventricle with pulmonary stenosis, and others. In Eisenmenger's syndrome (reversal of left to right shunts like VSD, ASD, PDA) also there occurs cyanosis. The differential cyanosis (toes are cyanosed, fingers are not) is typically noticed in PDA with reversal. Presence of clubbing with cyanosis invariably indicates central cyanosis.

HISTORY OF PAST ILLNESS

In a patient with cardiovascular disease the following past histories are likely to be significant.

Acute Rheumatic Fever

If the child suffered from rheumatic fever in childhood, he may suffer from various types of valvular heart diseases, mitral stenosis being the commonest. Very often there is a gap between the onset of rheumatic fever and development of symptoms of rheumatic heart disease (RHD). Following a single attack of rheumatic fever in childhood (5 to 15 years of age) symptoms of RHD develops in third or fourth decade. However, the patient may become symptomatic much earlier, even in the very first decade.

Ask for *migrating polyarthritis* in *childhood*. It should primarily affect the *big joints*. These inflamed joints are *very painful* so much so that the child has to be carried for toilet. Also, ask how many such episodes he has suffered, whether he has received penicillin prophylaxis or not? It should be kept in mind that a patient might be suffering from RHD, yet he may not give history of rheumatic fever. This is possible because if the major manifestations were not arthritis and chorea, the child or the parents may not be able to know that they had such an important illness. Also, remember that people often tell that there was rheumatic fever, but unless it fits into the criteria described above it should not be accepted easily (often rheumatic fever is overdiagnosed).

Hypertension

Ask if at any time he has/had been detected to be hypertensive. How to collect history of hypertension has been described elsewhere. Hypertension can subsequently cause or can be associated with left ventricular failure, coronary artery disease, hypertensive hypertrophic cardiomyopathy, dissecting aneurysm of aorta and co-arctation of aorta.

Diabetes Mellitus

History of diabetes mellitus is important in CVS because, it is a major risk factor for CAD. Diabetics may present atypically; as painless myocardial infarction or with diastolic dysfunction. Diabetics are also more prone to suffer from peripheral vascular disease.

Syphilis

Aortic regurgitation, aneurysm of ascending aorta and coronary ostial stenosis causing anginal pain are the cardiovascular manifestations of syphilis. Cardiovascular syphilis being a tertiary syphilis it takes fifteen to twenty years for its development after the exposure. How to collect history of syphilis has been described earlier.

Tuberculosis

The cardiac problems of tuberculosis are pericarditis, pericardial effusion and constrictive pericarditis. How to collect history of tuberculosis has been described too.

Chronic Respiratory Illnesses

There are several respiratory illnesses which can lead to cor pulmonale in later life. Most important among them is chronic bronchitis. Others are interstitial lung diseases, bilateral bronchiectasis, emphysema, gross deformity of the chest wall and so on.

Maternal Illnesses and Therapy

In case of suspected congenital heart disease major illnesses in the mother and drugs received during pregnancy have to be collected. Maternal systemic lupus erythematosus (SLE), Rubella are known to be associated with congenital heart diseases. Drugs in pregnancy which are known to cause foetal abnormality are anti-epileptic drugs and others.

Past History of Similar Illnesses

The cardiac illnesses which are likely to occur repeatedly are PSVT, episodes of congestive cardiac failure, angina of variable severity depending on the stage of CAD and cyanotic spells in TOF.

FAMILY HISTORY

Hypertension, coronary artery disease, sudden death, cardiomyopathy (particularly hypertrophic variety) can occur in many members of the family. So ask about these illnesses in the family. Few other genetically transmitted conditions which can be associated with cardiovascular abnormalities are Marfan's syndrome (AR, MR, and Aortic dilatation), Ehlers-Danlos syndrome (MR), Turner's syndrome (Coarctation of aorta, Bicuspid aortic valve), Friedreich's ataxia (cardiomyopathy and conduction defects), Muscular dystrophy (cardiomyopathy), etc.

PERSONAL HISTORY

Occupation	Sedentary workers—CAD
Smoking	CAD and peripheral vascular disease
Alcohol	CAD and Cardiomyopathy
IV drug addicts	Right-sided endocarditis

TREATMENT HISTORY

Treatment of cardiovascular diseases is often prolonged. Hence, enquire about the drugs the patient is already taking, because doubling of prescription may lead to dangerous complications (digoxin and anticoagulants). Drugs may alter the physical signs, even the investigations. For instance, if a patient is on digoxin, the heart rate may be slow in spite of heart failure, the pulse deficit may be less (<10) even if there is atrial fibrillation. ST segment changes may be due to drugs like digitalis (inverted check mark), or quinidine like anti-arrhythmic drugs (long QT). If the patient has already received antibiotics, blood culture may not show any growth of the organism in the setting of infective endocarditis. If the patient has received glucocorticosteroids ESR may become normal in spite of carditis. Many other non-cardiac drugs may have cardiac toxicity or may have drug interaction with cardiac drugs. Hence, details of the drugs being taken for prolonged period, drugs taken in recent past and the drugs being continued should be taken into account before prescribing drugs for any cardiac ailment. Treatment with repeated blood transfusion is also important as it is associated with Haemochromatosis leading to dilated cardiomyopathy.

MENSTRUAL HISTORY

Importance of menstrual history is same as in other conditions. There are some cardiac conditions where pregnancy should be avoided (already discussed). Institutional delivery may be recommended for some patients, surgical intervention may be needed for the cardiac condition in spite of pregnancy.

Radiological exposure should be avoided as far as possible. One thing should be remembered that in pregnancy there can be several cardiovascular alterations without any true cardiac illness. Also, remember that the criteria for the diagnosis of hypertension in pregnancy and in non-pregnant state are different.

It has been already discussed that three fourth of the diagnosis in a neurological case comes from history. If this has not been reached, history taking is incomplete. Patient may not complain everything of his own, he says what he feels important; but it is our duty to extract as much information as possible by tactful questioning and careful interpretation of the answers. The components of the diagnosis in a neurological case are:

1. Nature of the lesion
2. Structures affected
3. Site of the lesion
4. Aetiology (Cause).

NATURE OF THE LESION

Neurological disorders are classified into several groups like; cerebrovascular, degenerative, demyelinating, neoplastic (intracranial tumors), infective, deficiency disorders, etc. These disorders behave more or less in a predicted manner as regards their onset and course is concerned. Nature of the lesion can be decided on the basis of this clinical behavior. So in every case the exact mode of onset and the clinical course should be known. However, in acute neurological cases if the patient comes too early for consultation, it may not be possible to decide the course of the disease. Let us see how much information we get from the onset and course of the illness.

Gradual Onset and Progressive Course

- Degenerative disorders (Motor neuron disease, Parkinson's disease, Heredofamilial ataxia, nutritional toxin-mediated neuropathies)
- Space Occupying Lesions (SOL): Here in addition to neurological symptoms there will be features of raised intracranial pressure—headache, vomiting, papilloedema. There can be convulsions also.

Gradual Onset and Regressing Course (Tendency to Improve)

- Deficiency disorders: With replacement of the deficiency factor there will be improvement of the condition, improvement may be incomplete (Vitamin deficiency neuropathy, subacute combined degeneration of the cord).

Acute Onset and Worsening Course

- Cerebrovascular disease: particularly cerebral haemorrhage (can happen to thrombosis and embolism also).
- Infective disease: Tubercular meningitis, Encephalitis.

Acute Onset and Regressing Course

- Cerebrovascular disease: Thrombosis, Embolism, Haemorrhage: all can improve
- Demyelinating diseases
- Infective diseases: Pyogenic meningitis (tubercular meningitis and encephalitis can improve also). The most important feature of an infective disorder is it starts with fever. Fever can be present in intracerebral as well as in subarachnoid bleed, but it is never the starting complaint. In meningitis the sequence of events is fever, headache, vomiting and altered sensorium. In case of subarachnoid haemorrhage the sequence of events is headache, vomiting, altered sensorium and fever.

To decide the nature of the lesion this scheme works well in most of the situations, but there are exceptions too. For example, a CNS tumor may present as stroke due to bleeding into the tumor. A space occupying lesion (neoplastic lesion, granuloma or a cyst) may not have feature of raised intracranial tension, particularly if the SOL is a small one and it is situated in the supratentorial region. The middle-aged paraplegic form of multiple sclerosis may start gradually and have a progressive course, even if the nature of the lesion is demyelinating. Parkinson's disease may improve in the initial part of the course of the disease with treatment though it is basically a degenerative condition. A case of SOL may improve temporarily with anti-oedema measures. Febrile illness of any kind can precipitate a paralytic episode of multiple sclerosis mimicking an infective nature of the illness.

This protocol may not work well in spinal cord diseases (details later on).

STRUCTURES INVOLVED

From history one can fairly know the structures involved. The structures may be different parts of the brain like motor, sensory, various cranial nerves, bladder and bowel (autonomic), different parts of the brain (various lobes of the brain, cerebellum, etc). Let us see how we can know these structures from history.

Frontal Lobe

Focal motor seizures, weakness mostly monoplegia, deterioration in mental function, change in social behaviour, impairment of vision (due to compression of the optic nerve), impairment of sense of smell (due to involvement of the olfactory nerve) and speech defect.

Parietal Lobe

There may be sensory Jacksonian type of fits, sensory inattention on the opposite side of the body, asteriognosis (inability to recognize known objects in the affected hand in darkness or with eyes closed) and speech defects mostly receptive if the dominant parietal lobe is affected. Alexia and agraphia may be noticed in lesions of the dominant angular gyrus lesion. Apraxia, various forms of agnosia (particularly finger agnosia) and acalculia can also be seen. Lesion in the opposite angular gyrus can cause disorder in body image, so that the patient develops a tendency to neglect his affected one half of the body. This can be noticed in the form of dressing apraxia (he may forget to put on the dress on the affected side, may not be able to know right or left side of the dress). An abnormal type of movement disorder is noticed in parietal lobe lesion. Both in resting as well as in action athetoid movements of the affected hand may be noticed (pseudoathetosis). There may be visual field defects (quadrantic) due to involvement of the optic radiation. This is rarely complained by the patient, mostly revealed on examination.

Unless meticulously enquired parietal lobe lesions may be missed from history, and unless suspected in the history; casual examination may also miss these defects.

Temporal Lobe

Lesions in the temporal lobe causes more ill-defined symptoms and if not carefully listened may be passed away as hysterical or psychiatric in nature. Various types of hallucinations (like auditory, gustatory and olfactory) occur. There can occur uncinate fits (patient develops aura of smell or taste followed by involuntary movements involving lips, muscles of mastication, pharyngeal muscles). There can be perverted memory. Patient may feel unfamiliar things/events as familiar (*déjà vu* phenomenon) or familiar things/events may be felt as unfamiliar (*jamais vu* phenomenon). There can be visual field defects too (quadrantic). Emotional changes may be abrupt in onset can be noticed often taking the forms of panic attacks. Objects may appear smaller or larger, more distant or near than the real. Patient may describe his past life events, may complain of dreams of similar types coming repeatedly. There can be tinnitus, but hearing loss is uncommon. In lesion of the dominant temporal lobe there can be Wernicke's type of aphasia.

Occipital Lobe

Visual aura may precede convulsions. There can be visual field defects which may affect the way of living, so that the patient may hit the wall on the affected side. There can be several types of visual agnosia, like object agnosia, colour agnosia, prosopagnosia (inability to recognize face). Visual inattention is another specific feature of occipital lobe lesion. However, it may be difficult to detect occipital lobe lesion from history only.

Like this different parts of the brain have got some specific features which can be known from the history, details of which can be known from textbooks of neurology.

Cerebellar Lesions

In cerebellar lesions the patient complains of difficulty in walking/ unsteadiness of gait. This may be misunderstood as weakness of the limbs, so history should be collected carefully to understand what exactly the patient means. The patient may say that he is not able to put his feet in the desired place. In the upper limb he may say that there is tremulousness of the hands particularly in attempting to hold something or picking up some object. He may not be able to write clearly as he used to do it earlier, he may spill the water while attempting to drink particularly when the glass comes near the mouth. All these features may not be easy to conclude from the history. The other feature which can reveal that it is a cerebellar lesion is the defect in speech (while collecting history mark the type of speech). In cerebellar disorders speech becomes scanning means, syllables of a word get separated.

Often it is difficult to decide whether it is cerebellar parenchymal lesion or lesion is in the cerebellar connection. If the patient complains of truncal ataxia (patient will not be able to sit or stand steadily), it suggests lesion is in the vermix of the cerebellum, hence the primary cerebellar parenchymal lesion rather than its tract lesion. There are other signs which can be decided on examination only.

CRANIAL NERVES

- First cranial nerve: Patient complains of loss of sense of smell or perverted sense of smell. Unilateral lesion is rarely complained of, but it has got more pathological significance. There may be hysterical anosmia, where the patient not only refuses that he is not able to smell anything but also refuses to detect the irritating nature of ammonia (which is due to stimulation of the fifth nerve). This type of hysterical anosmia is found in cases of minor head injury where the victim wants to get better compensation.

- Second cranial nerve: Partial lesions in the optic nerve will cause blind spots in the visual field, but this may not be always noticed by the patient. More commonly patient complains of diminished visual acuity (both to near and distant objects). With progressive lesions of the optic nerve visual acuity diminishes in a progressive manner:
    - Inability to see small letters in a book or newspaper
    - Inability to see large letters
    - Inability to count fingers
    - Inability to appreciate hand movements
    - Inability to appreciate light

  Also, in the early stage of optic nerve lesion there may be poor appreciation of colour. One of the commonest cause of sudden blindness is disease of the optic nerve. Transient monocular blindness (a shade passing across the field of vision) may be a form of transient ischaemic attack (TIA) involving the ophthalmic artery. Pain on movement of the eyeball (in or behind the eye) suggests optic neuritis/retrobulbar neuritis.

- Third/ Fourth/Sixth cranial nerve: In lesions of these motor nerves of the eye there will be diplopia and squint (squint is often detected by the relatives). This squint can be utilized to know the presence of ophthalmoplegia in unconscious persons. There are several types of ophthalmoplegia; like supranuclear, nuclear, infranuclear and internuclear. Squint and diplopia are features of nuclear and infranuclear lesion. In supranuclear lesions there occurs conjugate deviation of the eyes without diplopia (This is also temporary). The other feature of third nerve involvement may be ptosis. In fact, diplopia may be masked by ptosis due to closure of the pupil. However, ptosis may be due to primary muscle disease (myasthenia gravis) or due to involvement of the sympathetic fibers. In third nerve lesion another symptom may be observed that is impaired vision particularly near vision (loss of accommodation) due to parasympathetic nerve involvement causing dilatation of the pupil.

- Fifth cranial nerve: In fifth nerve lesion there is impaired sensation over half of the face, so that the patient complains of numbness over the affected area. If there is loss of pain and temperature sensation also, he may complain that he is not able to appreciate the temperature of the water while washing his face, may say that he is not able to feel the hotness of the tea in the affected cheek. Due to involvement of the motor component he may say that there is deviation of the chin to one side (to the side of the paralysis) on attempt to protrude the mandible. There may be difficulty in chewing too.

- Seventh nerve: From history one can say whether it is was upper or lower motor neurone type of facial palsy. In lower motor neurone lesion eye remains open even during sleep (due to paralysis of the Orbicularis oculi) and the angle of the mouth is deviated to the opposite side (due to paralysis of the Orbicularis oris). In upper motor neurone lesion eyes are not affected. In some situations eyes are affected without affection of the mouth. This is possible in partial lesions involving the terminal fibers of the facial nerve (i.e. Leprosy). Remember that these facial asymmetries are often marked by the relatives first than the patient particularly the condition of the eye. The patient notices only when he sees his face in a mirror. However, the patient may complain of drooling of saliva or water from the angle of the mouth or involuntary dropping of lachrymal fluid from the affected eye.

• Eighth nerve: Unilateral 8th nerve lesion may not be easily revealed from history. Persistent tinnitus in a particular ear may suggest lesion in that side vestibulo-cochlear nerve. However, intelligent people can complain of diminished hearing in one ear. Invariably the lesion is in the infranuclear segment, because unilateral supranuclear lesion does not affect hearing. If the vestibular component is affected also there will be vertigo, but severe vertigo is not a feature of 8th nerve lesion rather it is due to involvement of the vestibular nucleus or its central connections. Tinnitus is another symptom of eighth nerve lesion. It rarely occurs in cortical lesions, but a noisy sound may be complained of, often taking the form of an auditory hallucination. Tinnitus occurs in lesions of the acoustic apparatus (cochlear/retrocochlear components).

• Ninth, Tenth cranial nerves: Truly lesions of these nerves are better revealed from history than from examination. The symptoms are dysphagia, dysphonia and dysarthria. Other evidences may be nasal regurgitation of food/water and nasal intonation of voice, induction of cough while taking food or drinks. Patient may have difficulty in swallowing his own saliva resulting in its accumulation in the throat. He may carry a spittoon/pot to collect his saliva. Relatives may complain that the patient is having excessive snoring and mouth breathing during sleep. Unilateral upper motor neurone lesion of these nerves does not cause any problem.

- Eleventh cranial nerve: Isolated eleventh cranial nerve lesion is uncommon. It is involved with the 9th and 10th cranial nerves; hence the symptoms are as described above. However, due to bilateral paralysis of the sternomastoid and the trapezius patient may not be able to keep the head straight. In sternomastoid paralysis (as in myotonic dystrophy) head tends to fall forward and in trapezius paralysis (motor neurone disease, poliomyelitis and myasthenia gravis) head tends to fall backward. There will be dropping of the shoulder on that side and he may complain of difficulty in lifting of the arm above the head.

- Twelfth nerve: There will be dysarthria (difficulty in uttering t and d) and deviation of the tongue to one side (to the paralyzed side). He may have difficulty in chewing food and in swallowing. In upper motor neurone lesions the tongue may appear small and stiff. Unilateral lesion does not affect articulation.

MOTOR SYSTEM

The motor system has got two parts; the upper motor neurone (UMN) and the lower motor neurone (LMN). The nerve cells in the motor cortex and its fibers (the corticospinal tract/pyramidal tract) constitute the upper motor neurone. The anterior horn cells, the anterior root and the motor peripheral nerve form the lower motor neurone. From history one can know whether it is UMN or LMN lesion. In both there will be weakness. If weakness is associated with atrophy (in patient's language it is thinning) of the limb/part it is likely to be LMN lesion. However, it takes a few weeks for atrophy to develop. Hence, it may not be possible to diagnose an acute LMN lesion from history only. The limb in LMN lesion is limp, so that he is not able to maintain any posture and there will be a wide range of passive movement around the affected joints. In UMN lesion the limb feels stiff so that there is a limited range of passive movement and more resistance to it. There may be an abnormal posture of the limb. Remember that in an acute UMN lesion (state of spinal shock) these features may be missing. In lower motor neurone lesion the other thing which the patient or the relatives may complain is flickering involuntary movements (fasciculation) in the affected muscles. Paraplegia, Monoplegia, Quadriplegia can be both due to UMN and LMN lesion. However, hemiplegia is mostly due to UMN lesion.

Another type of motor deficit occurs due to primary diseases of the muscles like myopathy and muscular dystrophy. Myopathy often affects a group of muscles (Limb girdle type, Facioscapulohumeral type, proximal type, etc.) and invariably it is symmetrical. No fasciculation is complained.

Motor weakness due to involvement of the peripheral nerve can occur, but most commonly there is sensory symptoms too, as most of the peripheral nerves are mixed nerves. However, there are a few neuropathies which affect predominantly motor fibers (lead neuropathy). In all these situations weakness and thinning (atrophy) starts from the peripheral parts and with the progress of the disease more and more proximal parts of the same muscle/ more proximal muscles are involved. In conditions like Peroneal muscular atrophy muscular atrophy progresses horizontally; initially in the lower limbs, later in the upper limbs also.

From history one can know which groups of muscles are affected. If the proximal muscles of the lower limbs are affected, patient will have difficulty in getting up from sitting posture. If he tries so, he will require support, at times his own legs (climbing his own body). In the upper limbs the patient will have difficulty in doing work above head like combing hairs or putting something on the shelves over head. If the distal muscles, say small muscles of the hands are affected, he will have problem in doing finer work like writing/ painting, etc. With involvement of the intrinsic muscles of the foot patient will face difficulty in walking on wet/ slippery/muddy surface.

The other part of the motor system is the extrapyramidal system. Here there will be changes in the tone (both hypertonia and hypotonia possible); so that the patient may say that his limbs are appearing to be stiff or limp. There may be various types of involuntary movements; commonest being tremor. The peculiarity of tremor due to extrapyramidal disorder is it occurs in the resting state involving the distal parts like fingers (tremor decreases on putting into action). Whatever may be described in words, it will be difficult to give full description of all the involuntary movements. Hence, students should see all varieties of involuntary movements and get acquainted with them. In addition to the involuntary movements, gait and postural abnormalities are other problems of extrapyramidal disorder, enquire about them.

SENSORY SYSTEM

Symptoms related to the sensory system are more vague and nonspecific. However, patient may complain of some positive symptoms like root pain or negative symptoms like numbness. It is very difficult to know the types of sensory abnormality from history only. Even examination may not yield satisfactory result in every case. Remember that sensory examination should be done when the patient is fully cooperative and relaxed, at times may take several sittings. Depending on the type of structure affected there will be different types of sensory findings. Some of them are:

- **Sensory loss in patches** (may be hypopigmented) Leprosy
- **Nerve type:** Sensory loss will be according to the distribution of the concerned nerve. For example, in ulnar nerve lesion there will be sensory loss in the medial side of the hand, in Median nerve lesion there will be loss of sensation on the lateral three and half fingers of the hand, in lesions of the Common Peroneal Nerve loss of sensation will be on the lateral aspect of the leg and on the dorsum of the foot. So one should have knowledge about sensory distribution of all major peripheral nerves.
- **Polyneuropathic type:** Here sensation will be impaired first in the distal parts; longer the peripheral nerve earlier it will be affected. In the lower limbs it will produce stocking type sensory loss and in the upper limbs it will cause gloves type sensory loss. All modalities are almost equally affected.

- **Root type:** There may be root pain. This is a burning, constricting or electric shock like pain which increases on coughing, sneezing and movements of the spine. Root pain can get relieved in a particular posture. Sensory loss will be along the distribution of the corresponding root. So one should have knowledge about dermatomal arrangement of the body. Again all modalities of sensation will be equally affected.

- **Tract type:** There are two main sensory tracts. The posterior column carries touch, vibration, position sense, etc. Lesion in this tract will produce sensory ataxia—means patient will have difficulty in walking in darkness or may have unsteadiness on closure of the eye. He may also tell that he does not feel anything below a particular level, if gross he may say that he does not feel whether he has cloth or not/ may say that he feels that his body has been divided below the particular level. To know whether the limbs are in correct position or not, he has to voluntarily move the limbs over a wider range. Similar thing may happen in lesions involving the upper limbs, so that the patient repeatedly moves the fingers to know their position (piano playing movements). The sensory level is more clearly described by the patient when it is over the trunk, but when it is on the limbs patient may not be able to tell (it is to be found out by examination). In lesions affecting the spinothalamic tract patient will not be able to feel pain or temperature sensation so that he might develop painless injuries/ ulcers, may develop blisters due to hot compression/burns due to cigarette buds.

Dissociated sensory loss is also a tract type sensory loss, where pain and temperature sensations are lost whereas posterior column types of sensations are preserved. This is seen in syringomyelia, intramedullary tumors, lateral medullary syndrome, etc.

- **Hemisensory loss:** Here sensation is lost over one half of the whole body (often all modalities equally) i.e. body as well as face. The lesion is in the region of internal capsule.

- **Hemisensory loss with thalamic over reaction:** In lesions of the thalamus in addition to the loss of sensation on half of the body, there is exaggerated appreciation of pain sensation on the affected side.

- **Cortical type of sensory loss:** Here primary sensations are intact. From history it will be difficult to know this type of sensory impairment. But asteriognosis may help. Very rarely the patient may say that holding an object on the affected hand he is not able to identify the object, but on transferring the object to the other hand he is promptly able to detect it (all of course either in darkness/eyes closed).

Asked meticulously and interpreted carefully a lot of information can be obtained from history about the sensory system.

SITE OF LESION

After knowing the structures affected one should know where they are affected. To determine the site of lesion one should have sound knowledge in neuroanatomy.

The major structures and their relative placement should be remembered. The anatomy of the spinal cord and brainstem at different levels, the basal ganglia, internal capsule cortical structure and functional representations, the cerebral arterial circulation and the venous circulations, the CSF (cerebrospinal fluid) pathway, intracranial and extracranial course of the cranial nerves, cerebellar anatomy and its connections root value and the course of the peripheral nerves all are important. Always attempt should be made to put the lesion at one place instead of putting multiple lesions.

Let us discuss some examples.

Example 1: A common structure affected in several neurological conditions is involvement of the corticospinal tract, presenting with motor weakness. The localization of the lesion will be as follows:

- Monoplegia with convulsion—Cerebral Cortex
- Monoplegia without convulsion—Corona radiata
- Hemiplegia with same side UMN Facial Palsy—Internal Capsule
- Cross hemiplegia—Brainstem lesion (Depending on the site, the corresponding motor cranial nerve will be affected. This cranial nerve paralysis will be LMN type and it will be on the opposite side of the limb weakness (same side of the lesion), hence cross hemiplegia
- Hemiplegia without any cranial nerve palsy—Spinal hemiplegia.

Example 2: If a patient has got seventh and eighth nerve lesion and cerebellar signs on the same side, the probable site of lesion is cerebellopontine angle (CP Angle).

Example 3: If a patient has got unilateral/ bilateral 3rd and/ or 4th nerve (even 6th nerve) with unilateral/ bilateral pyramidal sign, the probable site of lesion is interpeduncular fossa (as seen in Tubercular meningitis).

Example 4: If a patient has got unilateral 3rd, 4th and 6th nerve paralysis with numbness (sensory impairment) in the upper part of the same side face, the probable site of lesion is near the superior orbital fissure.

Example 5: If a patient has got proptosis and congestion of the eye and weakness of 3rd and 4th cranial nerve, numbness in the face (5th Nerve) on the same side, the probable site of lesion is near the cavernous sinus.

Example 6: If a case comes with paraplegia with thinning (atrophy) of the legs probably the lesion is below L1 vertebra (Cauda equina lesion); similarly if there is paraplegia without any complaint in the upper limb and without atrophy (thinning), the lesion is somewhere between T2 and L1. If there is quadriplegia/quadriparesis and it is a cord lesion (say there is bladder involvement) the site of lesion will be in the cervical cord. Quadriplegia with lower cranial nerve involvement/ cerebellar symptoms suggests high cervical cord compression.

Once the nature of the lesion, structures affected and the site of lesion are identified it is easy to reach at an aetiological diagnosis.

APPROACH TO A CASE WITH SPINAL CORD DISEASE

In a case with spinal cord disease the approach is little bit different. Let us first discuss how to suspect that it could be a primary spinal cord problem. The following points will help.

- If the complaints are solely confined to limbs without any symptoms of cranial nerve involvement or changes in the higher function (speech, consciousness, convulsion, memory etc).
- If bladder and bowel are affected.
- If there is history suggestive of root pain/tract pain.
- If the patient is able to appreciate a definite sensory level.
- If there is bony deformity of the spine and the complaints (whatever he has got) are confined to below that deformed spinal level.

However, it has to be kept in mind that there can be both spinal cord as well as intracranial lesions.

In a case with spinal cord problem it is required to differentiate whether it is a compressive or a non-compressive myelopathy. This is important because compressive lesions are basically curable conditions if operated in time. Hence, the decision has to be made quickly.

Features of Compressive Myelopathy

1. Most of the compressive myelopathies are gradual in onset and progressive in course except traumatic paraplegia, prolapse of the intervertebral disc, spinal epidural abscess/ haematoma, collapse of a vertebra (which may be due to Pott's spine, secondaries or multiple myeloma).
2. Presence of root pain. It is a type of pain which is appreciated along the distribution of the affected root; it is a burning, constricting or electric shock-like in character;

increases on coughing, sneezing and movement of the spine.

3. Presence of vertebral deformity and/or tenderness.

4. Sequential involvement of limbs or tracts. For example, one upper limb is affected first then lower limb of the same side then lower limb of the opposite side and opposite side upper limb is affected last. Similarly, it may start with motor weakness; later on develops sensory impairment and then bladder is affected.

5. Asymmetry of the lesion goes more in favour of compressive lesion. To start with non-compressive lesions may be asymmetrical also, but soon becomes symmetrical. Poliomyelitis and monomelic variety of motor neurone disease are asymmetrical even if they are non-compressive lesions.

6. If the patient is able to tell a sensory level, it is more likely to be compressive lesion. However, acute non-compressive lesion like transverse myelitis may have a level too.

In summary, it can be told that none of these features is diagnostic of compressive myelopathy; hence, all the points must be judiciously considered to reach at a conclusion. After deciding that it is a compressive lesion a probable level can be ascertained from the history also (see Example-6 under structures affected). However, an exact level can be known after examinations only.

PAST HISTORY IN A NEUROLOGICAL CASE

As in any other case, past history should include similar illness and significant illnesses. Neurological disorders which are likely to occur again and again (similar) are epilepsy, transient ischaemic attacks, multiple sclerosis, periodic paralysis, subarachnoid haemorrhage. Very rarely the neurological deficits of ADEM (Acute Disseminated Encephalomyelitis) can recur.

Significant past history depends on the type of neurological disorder. Let us discuss some examples.

- History of hypertension is significant in a case of CVA (Cerebrovascular Accident).
- History of TIA is significant in a case of CVA.
- History of rheumatic heart disease, recent myocardial infarction (mural thrombus) is important in a case of embolic stroke.
- In a suspected case of brain abscess history of CSOM (chronic suppurative otitis media), cyanotic congenital heart disease may be significant.
- History of syphilis is significant in several types of neurological problems.
- History of vaccination/viral infection in recent past is significant in ADEM. Acute post-infective polyneuropathy can also occur following viral infection.
- History of head injury may be important in a case of epilepsy.
- History of tuberculosis is significant in a suspected case of compressive myelopathy, tubercular meningitis, and multiple cranial nerve palsy.
- History of recent childbirth is important in a case with loss of consciousness with or without convulsion (could be puerperal cortical venous sinus thrombosis).

- Acute cerebellitis may occur in cases of chicken pox and typhoid fever.
- History of diabetes mellitus may be important in evaluating cases of metabolic encephalopathy and stroke.

And there are many more which one can know with progress in overall knowledge in neurology.

FAMILY HISTORY IN A NEUROLOGICAL CASE

The following conditions may occur in several members of a family. These conditions may be as follows:

Genetically Transmitted Conditions

- Muscular dystrophies
- Heredofamilial ataxias
- Different types of HSMN (Hereditary sensory motor polyneuropathy).
- Huntington's chorea

Remember that all the features may not manifest equally in all affected members of the family.

Familial Clustering Disorders

These are mostly nutritional toxin-mediated diseases like lathyrism, nutritional neuromyelopathies.

Even if there is no family history of similar illness present, history of consanguineous marriage in the family should be obtained. Autosomal recessive disorders can get manifested by this.

PERSONAL HISTORY

In a strictly vegetarian (vegan) vitamin B_{12} deficiency leading to subacute combined degeneration of the cord is possible.

A person working in a lead industry may suffer from lead neuropathy.

Sewerage workers may suffer from leptospiral meningitis. Recent change in bladder habit (hesitancy, urgency, incontinence, etc.) is highly significant in a neurological case. Bladder involvement may be the early sign of intramedullary lesion and is the late feature of extradural cord compression. Bladder affection is often (not always) a feature of completeness of a spinal cord lesion. If this is in the setting of compressive lesion, early surgical intervention is required. Unilateral corticospinal tract lesion does not affect the bladder (if at all transient). In conditions of dementia and in frontal lobe lesion there may be decline in social behaviour so that patient may pass urine where he is not supposed to do under normal situation. Similarly in a recovering spinal cord disease bladder may be the last to recover.

TREATMENT HISTORY

Treatment history is important under certain situations; like-
- Treatment status of hypertension and diabetes mellitus is required in evaluating an unconscious patient.
- Discontinuation of antiepileptic drugs may precipitate status epilepticus.
- Consumption of certain drugs can cause polyneuropathy, optic neuritis and auditory neuropathy.

- If it is a partially treated case, one has to remember that the physical signs, even investigations may get modified (partially treated pyogenic meningitis, tubercular meningitis, etc.).
- In recurring neurological problem like epilepsy one should know the response to previous treatment so that one can plan the future management.

History in Respiratory Disorders

> *Never be miser in using the xylocaine jelly,*
> *for catheterizing the bladder.*

The components of diagnosis in a respiratory case are:
1. **Pathological** (like consolidation/fibrosis/collapse, etc.)
2. **Anatomical** (like upper lobe/lower lobe/pleural, etc.)
3. **Aetiological** (like bacterial/fungal/neoplastic, etc.)

If possible respiratory functional status can be added to these components of diagnosis; means whether there is any compromise in the primary functions of the respiratory system, i.e. oxygen and carbon dioxide exchange?

History gives maximum information in a respiratory case, more than in a neurological case. History is more important in a respiratory case because very often the physical findings are confusing and misleading. A case with respiratory disease may present with the following complaints singly or in combinations. These are:
1. Cough (with/without sputum production)
2. Dyspnoea

3. Chest pain
4. Haemoptysis
5. Fever.

COUGH

Cough is the single most important complaint of respiratory diseases. Rarely it is noticed in diseases elsewhere. It is a protective reflex. It tries to keep the respiratory tract clean. Cough may be associated with sputum production or it may be dry. Dry cough suggests disease is in the upper respiratory tract or in the pleura. However, there can be dry cough in early parenchymal disease as in congestive stage of pneumonia and in interstitial lung diseases. It may be dry in early stage of bronchial tree disease like early stage of bronchogenic carcinoma and smoker's cough. Cough may be apparently dry in children and women as they often swallow the sputum. Cough with sputum production suggests lesion in the lower respiratory tract (below the vocal cords); it may be in the bronchial tree or in the lung parenchyma (part of the lung distal to the terminal bronchiole). The type of sputum produced helps in the diagnosis. Always try to see sputum yourself. The different types of sputum which can be encountered are:

a) Purulent: Here the sputum is thick and pus like. Such sputum is seen in lung abscess, bronchiectasis and amoebic liver abscess communicating to the lungs. In the latter condition the sputum is anchovy sauce type and the patient may be able to tell that there is flavour of liver when it is expectorated.

b) Mucopurulent: Sputum is a mixture of mucus and pus; seen in acute exacerbation of chronic bronchitis, also can be seen in tuberculosis.

c) Mucoid: Sputum is mucus type, typically seen in chronic simple bronchitis.

d) Rusty sputum: Sputum is uniformly mixed with small amount of RBCs as happens in the state of red hepatization of pneumonia.

e) Black sputum: Seen in coal workers, can be seen following exposure to smoky environment.

f) Frothy sputum: Seen when there is lot of water/ watery secretion in the lungs. This occurs in cases of Drowning and Organophosphorus poisoning. Pink frothy sputum is characteristic of pulmonary oedema.

g) Red currant jelly sputum: Seen in Klebsiellar pneumonia (jelly-like sputum mixed with blood).

In addition to the type of sputum produced some **other characters** of the sputum may help in the diagnosis. Profuse sputum is seen in lung abscess, bronchiectasis, pulmonary oedema (always ask the patient to collect the 24 hours sputum). Foul smelling sputum is seen in lung abscess, bronchiectasis. In these conditions sputum may not be foul smelling always as it is dependent on the presence of anaerobic organisms.

Timing of cough also helps in diagnosis. In chronic bronchitis, pulmonary tuberculosis and bronchiectasis cough is more marked in the morning. In chronic bronchitis cough is more marked in the winter season. Patient coughs vigorously but brings out only little amount of sputum (tenacious sputum). Cough and sputum production is often more marked in a particular body position in lung abscess and bronchiectasis. At times cough is increased in lying down posture and relieved in upright posture as in left ventricular failure. This may also be seen in mediastinal tumor and diaphragmatic hernia. In the former cough may be associated with dyspnoea. (There was a case of large amoebic liver abscess who was having persistent cough in lying down posture so much so that he was not able to sleep; for which he had to sit the whole night. This cough was relieved after aspiration of pus from the liver. This was because there had been a small leak of the abscess to the lung and the leakage was only in lying down posture; and no leakage in upright posture. After aspiration the liver tissue grew and sealed the leak.) Patients of chronic pharyngitis and nasal obstruction often cough more at night.

Smoker's cough typically increases after smoking. Cough which only comes on deglutition is seen in patients with lower cranial nerve palsy and tracheo-oesophageal fistula.

Character of cough can also help in diagnosis. At times only by listening to the cough it is possible to clinch the diagnosis. Bovine cough indicates paralysis of the vocal cords. Here the explosive nature of the cough is lost. Following a prolonged bout of cough a child takes a long noisy inspiration (whoop) is diagnostic of whooping cough. In pleurisy attempt to take deep inspiration or to cough causes pain so that the patient becomes afraid of coughing forcefully; but due to the underlying disease he has to cough. Here he suppresses the violent nature of the cough. This type of cough is often called a suppressed cough, which is typically seen in pneumonia with pleurisy. Hysterical cough is loud and barking; often it starts abruptly. Abrupt onset of a cough (may be associated with dyspnoea) in a child may be due to foreign body aspiration. Brassy cough (metallic tinge to the cough) may be due to compression of the major airway from outside. Paroxysmal cough may be a variant of bronchial asthma.

DYSPNOEA

Dyspnoea primarily occurs in diseases of the respiratory or cardiovascular system.

Dyspnoea due to respiratory diseases can be long standing or may be of short duration.

The causes of long duration dyspnoea are bronchial asthma, chronic bronchitis, emphysema and interstitial lung diseases. History can reveal the cause in most of these cases.

Dyspnoea of Long Duration

- If it is episodic in nature and associated with wheezing— Bronchial asthma.
- If it is persistent without wheezing—Interstitial lung disease.
- Persistent with wheezing—Perennial bronchial asthma. So the *outstanding feature of asthma is wheezing.*
- Dyspnoea associated with cough and sputum production— Chronic bronchitis.

In pure emphysema there is no sputum production. But often chronic bronchitis and emphysema coexist. In chronic bronchitis cough and sputum production occur earlier than dyspnoea (at times years before). Dyspnoea in chronic bronchitis may mimic the episodic nature of bronchial asthma due to acute exacerbation of the disease. *Hallmark of chronic bronchitis is sputum production.*

Dyspnoea of Short Duration

There are some situations where dyspnoea is of a few hours/ days in duration. Such causes are:

- Collapse
- Pneumothorax
- Pulmonary infarction
- Diaphragmatic/ Intercostal paralysis
- Pneumonia involving more than one lobe
- Massive pleural effusion
- Major airway obstruction even without causing collapse

In most of these conditions dyspnoea is maximum at the beginning except in tension pneumothorax (not in closed or open pneumothorax), massive pleural effusion and major airway obstruction. Because the lost lung function is taken up by the healthy lung within some days, severity of dyspnoea tends to decrease with the progress of time. In massive pleural effusion and in tension pneumothorax as long as fluid or air is going on accumulating in the pleural space dyspnoea will go on increasing. In cases of major airway obstruction if the obstruction is increasing in nature (growth) dyspnoea may increase, if it is regressing in nature (mucus plug) dyspnoea may decrease. However, the most important feature of major airway obstruction is stridor (noisy inspiration). Similarly if the intercostal paralysis progresses and involves the diaphragm (ascending paralysis) dyspnoea may increase. If the diaphragmatic paralysis is due to compression of the phrenic nerve, dyspnoea will decrease with the progress of time.

There are some situations where dyspnoea may be of neither long (years) nor short duration (days); it may be in terms of months. This may be seen in initial stage of bronchial asthma, or initial stages of other diseases enumerated in the list of causes of long-standing dyspnoea. However, one cause typically falls in this category is pulmonary eosinophilia.

HAEMOPTYSIS

True haemoptysis is coughing out of blood from the lower respiratory tract. Always try to differentiate from haematemesis and spurious haemoptysis (discussed elsewhere). The common causes of haemoptysis are as follows.

Respiratory Causes

- Tuberculosis
- Bronchogenic carcinoma
- Bronchiectasis
- Lung abscess
- Chronic bronchitis
- Pulmonary infarction
- Bronchial adenoma
- Pulmonary AV malformation
- Fungal infection of the lungs

Non-respiratory Causes

Haemoptysis can occur in non-respiratory cases like mitral stenosis, primary pulmonary hypertension, Eisenmenger's syndrome, Tetralogy of Fallot, etc.

In primary bleeding disorders like thrombocytopenic conditions there can also be haemoptysis. Haemoptysis with features of glumerulonephritis suggests Goodpasture's syndrome.

Associated symptoms with haemoptysis can suggest the cause. For example-

- Cough, fever, weight loss with haemoptysis—Pulmonary tuberculosis. (Remember in pulmonary tuberculosis irrespective of the clinical findings X-ray is invariably abnormal but in endobronchial tuberculosis there can be clear X-ray. These cases mostly present with haemoptysis). Also remember that haemoptysis can occur in healed tuberculosis.

- Long history of profuse and purulent sputum, now having haemoptysis—Bronchiectasis.

- Short history of profuse purulent sputum, now having haemoptysis—Lung abscess.

- Frank haemoptysis with weight loss(may be a smoker)— could be Bronchogenic carcinoma.

- Repeated haemoptysis without deterioration in health (usually young female, often small in amount)—Bronchial adenoma.

- Repeated haemoptysis without deterioration in health (can be massive)—Pulmonary AV malformation.

- Sudden onset of dyspnoea followed by haemoptysis (often in a bedridden patient)—Pulmonary infarction.
- Dyspnoea on exertion with haemoptysis—Could be Mitral Stenosis.
- Haemoptysis in a case with Cyanotic heart disease—Could be TOF, Eisenmenger's syndrome.
- Long-standing cough with expectoration and haemoptysis (blood-streaked sputum)—Chronic Bronchitis.
- Pneumonic onset followed by red current jelly sputum—Klebsiellar pneumonia.
- If there is bleeding from other sites with haemoptysis—Bleeding/clotting disorder.

If a patient has got a long-standing underlying lung disease and the patient develops haemoptysis off and on, one should not simply tell that the cause of haemoptysis is due to the underlying lung disease. Bronchogenic carcinoma may be missed in early stage in the setting of chronic bronchitis (both occur in smokers), Fungal infection (for example, Aspergilosis) may be missed in a case of tuberculosis. In fact, it has been advised that every episode of haemoptysis should be evaluated as a fresh case.

FEVER

Fever as in any other case usually indicates infective in origin. High fever occurs in inflammation of the lung parenchyma (pneumonia). Also can occur in empyema thoracis and in lung abscess. A single shaking chill with high fever associated with cough (with/without pleuritic chest pain, with/without sputum) suggests pneumonia (so-called pneumonic onset).

Low-grade fever can occur in upper respiratory infection and infection in the bronchial tree (Bronchitis). There may not be fever in both these conditions. Irregular fever occurs in pulmonary tuberculosis. In tuberculosis fever can persist for months. In fact, one of the commonest causes of Pyrexia of unknown origin in a tropical country like ours is tuberculosis. Fever may be more marked in the evening.

Fever can occur in pulmonary infarction, but it occurs late; never is the starting complaint.

CHEST PAIN

The only pain sensitive structure in the respiratory system is the parietal pleura.

So pain due to diseases of the respiratory system has to involve the parietal pleura.

This type of pain is called pleuritic chest pain. The feature of pleuritic chest pain is it increases on deep inspiration and on coughing. It is a localized pain (often the patient points to the site of pain with a finger). If pleurisy proceeds to the development of pleural effusion, pain subsides. Similarly, in a case of pleural effusion after aspiration of pleural fluid pain may recur due to both pleural surfaces coming on contact with each other and rubbing.

Other causes of chest pain are either due to cardiovascular conditions (discussed elsewhere) or due to diseases of the chest wall. Diseases of the chest wall causing pain are trauma, fracture of a rib, metastatic deposits on the rib (secondary/multiple myeloma), infective conditions of the skin, costo-chondritis, etc. The hallmark of a chest wall pain is it is associated with tenderness. However, there are some non-chest wall conditions which can be associated with tenderness are empyema and amoebic liver abscess. Here I want to emphasize that in all cases of lower chest pain exclude intra-abdominal condition and in all cases of upper abdominal pain exclude intrathoracic condition.

Chest pain may be referred in origin as seen diseases involving the nerve roots (Herpes Zoster, vertebral diseases and extramedullary tumors).

PAST HISTORY

As usual in past history similar illnesses and significant illnesses should be collected.

Respiratory illnesses which can occur repeatedly are bronchial asthma, acute exacerbations of chronic bronchitis, acute infections in bronchiectasis, fibrocystic disease. There are a few other situations where repeated respiratory infections can occur. These are mitral stenosis, left to right shunt (ASD, VSD, and PDA), splenectomized individuals, AIDS, congenital agammaglobulinemia, multiple myeloma, diabetes mellitus, etc.

The respiratory infection may be in the form of bronchitis or pneumonia. There are some underlying lung conditions which can predispose to repeated attacks of pneumonia in the same segments, as seen in bronchiectasis and bronchial growth.

Sometimes pneumothorax can occur repeatedly.

Some general conditions like AIDS, Diabetes mellitus, prolonged glucocorticoid therapy predisposes the individual to suffer from tuberculosis. In some respiratory conditions like silicosis and chronic bronchitis also tuberculosis is more frequently seen.

In a suspected case of lung abscess history of loss of consciousness (epileptic fits/alcohol intoxication), surgery under general anaesthesia are important. In suspected cases of bronchiectasis history of measles or whooping cough in childhood may be significant.

FAMILY HISTORY

Genetically transmitted conditions of the respiratory system are few.

Alfa 1 anti-trypsin deficiency causing emphysema is one such disease. Bronchial asthma can occur in many members of the family though the exact mode of transmission is uncertain. Being air borne in nature, tuberculosis can affect many members of the family.

PERSONAL HISTORY

Significant personal history in a respiratory case are:

Smoking—chronic bronchitis, bronchogenic carcinoma

Alcohol—Aspiration pneumonia, tuberculosis

Extramarital sexual contact—AIDS and related respiratory illnesses

Housing condition—may help in ascertaining a precipitating factor of bronchial asthma.

History in Gastrointestinal Disorders

> *If in the same patient there is anaemia and hypoproteinemia, mostly the cause is in the gastrointestinal tract.*

Very little information is obtained from examination of the patients with diseases of the gastrointestinal (GI) system. Temporal profile of the illness is extremely important to reach at a diagnosis in these cases. Hence, history is of outmost importance in gastrointestinal disorders. The common symptoms of GI disorders are:

- Abdominal pain
- Abdominal swelling
- Vomiting
- Dysphagia
- Diarrhoea and constipation
- Jaundice
- Haematemesis (vomiting of blood)

- Melaena/haematochezia
- Bleeding per anum
- Weight loss

ABDOMINAL PAIN

Abdominal pain is a common complaint in clinical practice. There can be acute and chronic painful conditions. Acute painful abdominal conditions are more common and it needs sound power of clinical judgment for coming to a conclusion in such situations. These conditions not only give pain to the patient but also improper approach and treatment may lead to fatal outcome or may lead to unnecessary surgery. In acute abdominal conditions history gives maximum information and often can clinch the diagnosis. Time spent for an accurate history is never wasted. Rather there are instances where valuable time has been wasted for investigations and the patient dies due to delay in surgery (at times on the investigation table). In less clear-cut cases history should be taken and examinations have to be done repeatedly while the patient is on conservative treatment or being investigated. If investigations are done without reaching at a provisional diagnosis from history and examinations; the later may completely confuse the clinical set up. For example, if a case comes with clinical picture suggestive of acute appendicitis and an abdominal ultrasound is done early (when there may not be any evidence of appendicitis sonographically) and if it shows stones in the gallbladder the case may be treated as acute cholecystitis (though the stones may be silent and only accidentally detected).

ACUTE ABDOMINAL PAIN

While evaluating a case with abdominal pain a few things must be kept in mind. These are:

- Abdominal pain may not be due to abdominal conditions. It is the rule that in all cases of upper abdominal pain exclude the possibility of an intrathoracic condition like myocardial infarction or diaphragmatic pleurisy. Pain of nerve root origin can also be felt on the abdomen.
- Abdominal pain does not mean disorders of the GI tract or the related structures like liver, gallbladder, etc. may be due to structures of the genitourinary system.
- Possibility of occlusion of the intra-abdominal blood vessels
- Menstrual history in a female case should not be missed.
- All acute abdominal conditions need not be surgical. A few conditions like acute intermittent porphyria, lead poisoning, Henoch-Schönlein purpura, acute metabolic conditions like diabetic ketoacidosis and uraemia, gastric crisis of tabes dorsalis, sickle cell crisis, etc. can present as acute abdomen.

While collecting history the things to be clarified are:

- Type of pain
- Site of pain and its radiation
- Bladder and bowel
- Associated symptoms

Colicky Type of Pain

Obstruction to hollow viscus with limited distensibility causes colicky type of abdominal pain. This pain is of abrupt onset, quickly reaches a peak and abruptly subsides. During the peak of the pain the patient becomes restless, may roll over, may press something (like pillow) on the abdomen, and may tie something (like a piece of cloth) on the abdomen. Classically there are two types of colicky pain, i.e. intestinal colic and ureteric colic. Small intestinal colic is referred to periumbilical region and large intestinal colic is referred to hypogastric area. Though intestinal colic is commonly due to intestinal obstruction but it can be due to exaggerated peristaltic movement also. This is the mechanism of colicky pain in lead poisoning and in acute intermittent porphyria. In ureteric colic pain starts from loin radiates to groin and medial side of upper part of thigh and to the genitals (scrotum/ labia majora).

There are a few other situations where even if there is obstruction to hollow viscera there does not occur typical colicky pain. These are obstruction of ureter at pelvi ureteric junction, biliary tract obstruction and obstruction of urinary bladder at bladder neck. Obstruction at pelvi ureteric junction causes persistent pain (so-called renal colic) at renal angle. Hence renal colic is not a true colic. Biliary tract obstruction particularly obstruction to common bile duct of acute onset can cause colicky type of pain (biliary colic), but commonly it causes dull aching pain in right hypochondrium which may be referred to inferior angle of right scapula. Similarly, obstruction of the cystic duct causes constant type of pain in the right hypochondrium. Chronic obstruction to the biliary tract may not be painful at all (as in obstruction due to carcinoma head of pancreas). Obstruction to bladder neck causes retention of urine causing fullness of the bladder. If sensory system is intact it causes a constant aching pain in the suprapubic region. In a patient with impaired level of consciousness this may be the cause of persistent restlessness. Though intestinal obstruction causes pain gastric outlet obstruction does not cause pain, rather vomiting becomes the prominent complaint.

Persistent Abdominal Pain

This may be of two types; localized or diffuse.

Localized

Persistent localized pain is due to inflammation of the viscera, as in hepatitis, cholecystitis, pancreatitis, appendicitis, etc. The pain will be felt over the organ involved or over the corresponding dermatome when the surrounding parietal peritoneum is not affected. Once the adjacent parietal peritoneum is involved pain will be felt over the inflamed area. For example, in acute appendicitis initial pain will be felt in the umbilical area and it shifts to the right iliac fossa. This will be associated with tenderness and rigidity. Though the rigidity cannot be complained by the patient, tenderness can be marked by the patient. However, both these features are to be confirmed by examination.

In hepatitis pain is due to stretching of its capsule. This occurs if the stretching is over a short period as noticed in acute hepatitis and congestive heart failure. Gradual stretching does not cause pain as in fatty liver or carcinoma of the liver. A peculiar character of pain is felt in amoebic liver abscess.

Here pain is exaggerated on jerky movement so that the patient is afraid of walking briskly and often he walks by putting his hand over the liver (supporting the liver).

Pain of acute pyelonephritis is a deep seated abdominal pain, but the patient primarily complains of pain in the renal angle (angle between the 12th rib and erector spinae muscle).

Pain of acute pancreatitis is felt in the epigastric and umbilical region and is referred to back which is exacerbated on lying supine and partly relieved on sitting up with trunk bending forward. Pain of acute cholecystitis is felt in the epigastric area or over right hypochondrium, may be referred to right shoulder.

Diffuse

Persistent and diffuse abdominal pain is due to acute peritonitis. This may be due to several reasons. Some common causes are:

  i. Perforation of hollow organs like:
   - Peptic ulcer
   - Enteric perforation
   - Inflamed appendix
   - Gangrenous segment of strangulated intestine
   - Caecum in large gut obstruction and so on.
 ii. Rapture of other viscera like:
   - Amoebic liver abscess communicating to peritoneum
   - Gallbladder causing biliary peritonitis
   - Spleen leaking blood into the peritoneum
   - Ectopic pregnancy leaking blood into the peritoneum
   And so on.

If the content discharged into the peritoneum is infected (amoebic liver abscess, colonic content), inflammation will be severe than when the content which is noninfective. Leakage of blood and bile will cause less severe inflammation. Leakage of gastric content (highly acidic) and pancreatic enzymes as in acute pancreatitis will cause severe inflammation. Sudden leakage will cause more severe inflammation than gradual leakage.

Once there is peritonitis there will be diffuse tenderness and rigidity of the anterior abdominal wall. The pain and tenderness will increase on any sort of movement. Hence, the patient prefers to lie down quietly. Such patients when asked to sit will do so at their own comfort; avoiding any type of help. Sneezing and coughing also increases pain.

It is to be remembered that earlier two types of pain (colicky and localized persistent) can end up in diffuse persistent abdominal pain with the development of peritonitis.

Referred Pain

The other type of pain which is felt on the abdomen is referred pain. Here none of the abdominal organs is involved. The common causes are intrathoracic conditions like ischaemic myocardial pain (unstable angina/myocardial infarction), diaphragmatic pleurisy. Irritation of the nerve roots (T-7 to L-1) causes pain on the anterior abdominal wall along the distribution of the corresponding nerve root. Neuralgic pain along the distribution of one or few dermatome can be felt in Herpes Zoster. This may be really difficult to know in the early pre-eruptive stage of the condition.

Pain on the Abdominal Wall

Diseases affecting the abdominal wall can also cause abdominal pain. It may be a haematoma (on rectus sheath) or a parietal abscess. Here the pain is localized and it may be associated with localized swelling and tenderness. Throbbing character suggests abscess.

Vascular Pain

Vascular pain may be due to occlusion of the mesenteric artery or due to rupture of the abdominal aortic aneurysm. Though these conditions are mostly catastrophic in onset, but at times it can be more gradual in onset also. Patient may complain of mild abdominal pain for a few days before the sudden severe pain associated with circulatory collapse. In mesenteric artery occlusion there can be bloody diarrhoea. Pain is usually diffuse type but initially it can be colicky type also. In rupture of the abdominal aortic aneurysm pain will be referred to the sacral area and perineum. A type of pain occurs in atherosclerotic narrowing of the mesenteric artery called abdominal angina. Here pain starts fifteen to thirty minutes after intake of food and persists for several hours in the postprandial state.

Though from the features of the pain only one can predict the diagnosis, but the associated symptoms give maximum lead to reach at a diagnosis.

Fever: High fever with chill occurs in perinephric abscess and acute pyelonephritis. Fever with chill also occurs in cholangitis. Fever not necessarily high also occurs in acute cholecystitis, acute appendicitis and inflammatory conditions of other intra-abdominal organs. Fever for some days (two to three weeks) followed by diffuse abdominal pain suggests the possibility of enteric perforation.

Jaundice: Occurs in hepatitis and cholangitis. Intermittent fever, abdominal pain and jaundice (Charcot's biliary triad) suggests cholangitis. In hepatitis by the time jaundice appears fever subsides.

Haematuria: Ureteric colic associated with haematuria suggests stone in the urinary tract. Sometimes passage of clots can have similar pictures (clot colic).

Circulatory collapse: Abdominal pain followed by circulatory collapse suggests the possibility of splenic rupture, rupture of ectopic pregnancy, mesenteric artery occlusion, rupture of abdominal aortic aneurysm. If the pain is in the upper abdomen exclude myocardial infarction.

Amenorrhoea, abdominal pain, shock: In early pregnancy ruptures of ectopic pregnancy and in late pregnancy abruptio placentae should be thought of. In both conditions, there may or may not be vaginal bleeding. Of course, vaginal bleeding further helps in the diagnosis. But the combination of amenorrhoea, abdominal pain and vaginal bleeding commonly suggests abortion.

Strangury: Suggests stone is near the vesicoureteric junction, can be a feature of pelvic peritonitis. It is painful straining for passing urine, often with passage of little amount of urine.

Vomiting: Vomiting frequently accompanies many acute abdominal conditions. So vomiting may not help always. If the vomiting is projectile, it may suggest intestinal obstruction. Vomiting is often persistent in intestinal obstruction and in acute pancreatitis; however, in acute appendicitis vomiting occurs only for a few occasions at the onset. In the setting of intestinal obstruction, vomiting occurs early if the site of obstruction is in the proximal part, late if the obstruction is in the ileum or in the large gut. The sequence of events in small gut obstruction is pain-vomiting-abdominal distension; in large gut obstruction it is pain-distension-vomiting.

Bowel: In all cases of acute abdomen enquire about the bowel habit. Marked constipation for some days may later on present with features of intestinal obstruction. If the history is taken meticulously, it will be revealed that constipation occurred much before the onset abdominal pain. In these settings manual removal or an enema will solve the problem and can avert an unnecessary surgery (I have seen a few such cases). Absolute constipation (no passage of flatus or stool) occurs in both dynamic as well as adynamic obstruction. However, there can be a few motions at the onset, till the distal segment is evacuated. Red currant jelly stool (stool containing only mucus and blood) may be seen in cases of intussusception. Bloody diarrhoea in the setting of acute abdomen suggests mesenteric artery occlusion.

I have seen a female case with colicky abdominal pain with swelling of the abdomen being misdiagnosed as intestinal obstruction, though she was in labour pain. So what I want to emphasize is that in every female case with abdominal pain menstrual history is mandatory and always a pregnancy-related condition should be excluded, which may be abortion, labour (premature/term), rupture of ectopic pregnancy, abruptio placentae.

CHRONIC ABDOMINAL PAIN

Though there are several causes of acute abdomen, chronic abdominal pain occurs in limited conditions. These are some of the examples.
• Acid peptic disease
• Chronic pancreatitis
• Chronic cholecystitis
• Diverticulitis
• Irritable bowel syndrome (IBS)
• Subacute intestinal obstruction

In cases of acute abdomen examination of the patient reveals some valuable findings, but in chronic abdominal painful conditions examination of the patient does not show many findings. Hence, one has to depend more on the history to reach at a conclusion. It has to be remembered that the so-called pain in these conditions may not be truly painful; it may be a sense of discomfort. The following aspects are to be clarified to reach at a diagnosis.

Site of Pain

• Epigastric or slightly to the right of epigastric area—duodenal ulcer
• Epigastric or slightly to the left of epigastric area—gastric ulcer

- Right hypochondrium nearer to the costal margin—chronic cholecystitis.
- Diffuse/central abdominal pain—subacute intestinal obstruction (may be tubercular).
- Hypogastric region/left iliac fossa—diverticulitis/IBS.

Relationship to Food

- Food relieves pain—duodenal ulcer
- Food brings on pain—gastric ulcer
- Intolerance to fatty food—chronic cholecystitis/chronic pancreatitis.

Timing of Pain

- Pain occurring in late hours of night or early morning—duodenal ulcer
- Pain which is often diffuse starting fifteen to thirty minutes after intake of food and lasts for several hours suggests abdominal angina (Chronic mesenteric ischaemia).

Vomiting

- Induced vomiting (by putting finger into the throat)—Gastric ulcer
- Voluminous projectile vomiting suggests gastric outlet obstruction. However, in conditions of gastric outlet obstruction pain is rarely present possibly with the exception of pylorospasm due to an active duodenal ulcer. In other situations there can be a sense of discomfort (often sense of fullness).

- Intermittent vomiting is possible in subacute intestinal obstruction.

Appetite

True anorexia occurs in carcinoma of stomach, but it rarely causes pain unless it infiltrates into the posterior abdominal wall. However, dyspepsia to fatty food occurs in gallbladder diseases. Dyspepsia to protein-rich food occurs in carcinoma stomach. In gastric ulcer appetite is preserved, but patient may be afraid of taking food as food increases pain. In mesenteric ischaemia large meals cause more pain for which patient prefers to take small food at a time.

Fever

Abdominal pain with fever is seen in cholangitis, may be seen in abdominal tuberculosis.

Weight Loss

Chronic abdominal pain associated with weight loss may be seen in malignant conditions, abdominal tuberculosis, due to exocrine pancreatic insufficiency in patients with chronic pancreatitis, at times in chronic mesenteric ischaemia.

Bowel

Alternate constipation with diarrhoea occurs in intestinal tuberculosis and in irritable bowel syndrome. In abdominal tuberculosis there will be weight loss, in IBS this does not occur.

ABDOMINAL SWELLING

If a patient comes with complaint of abdominal swelling, enquire whether it is localized or generalized. A localized swelling (often complained as a mass) later on can behave like a generalized swelling. Hence, ask from which site it started. Depending on the site of origin of the swelling one can predict the organ from which it might have arisen. For example:

- From epigastric area—stomach, left lobe of liver
- From right hypochondrium—right lobe of the liver, gall-bladder
- From left hypochondrium—spleen
- From lumbar region—kidney, colon
- From right iliac fossa—Caecum, appendix, ovary
- Left iliac fossa—sigmoid colon, ovary
- Hypogastric region—bladder, uterus, ileum.

Lymph nodes can form a swelling almost anywhere. Any of these organs if hugely enlarged can occupy almost the whole abdomen and can mimic a generalized abdominal swelling.

In case of truly generalized abdominal swelling (abdominal protuberance) the patient will not be able to tell from which site it started. The causes of such abdominal protuberance are fat, flatus, faeces, fluid and in female foetus.

Fat rarely causes problem as often it is not complained of. If at all, it will be over a prolonged period and it will be part of the whole body obesity.

Flatus causes abdominal protuberance (distension) in the setting of intestinal obstruction (both dynamic and adynamic), acute dilatation of stomach and toxic megacolon. In all these situations the total clinical picture will be so obvious that it will be rarely a diagnostic problem.

Faeces causing abdominal swelling are similarly rare. The causes are congenital megacolon, a problem of early childhood. Acquired megacolon can be seen in adult and at times it is due to myxoedema and Chagas' disease. The outstanding accompanying complaint will be marked and prolonged constipation.

Foetus causing abdominal swelling is often obvious. History of amenorrhoea in the childbearing age group is the most important accompanying complaint. Other signs of pregnancy may also be there. Though it is invariably obvious, but at times it can put the doctor in a delicate situation. Pregnancy in an unmarried girl or in a widow may not be accepted by the guardians easily, particularly in our society. I have seen parents charging the doctor under such situations. So one should be tactful in dealing with such situations; better it will be to ask for a documentary evidence for this like a pregnancy test in urine or an ultrasound.

The commonest cause of generalized abdominal swelling is fluid (ascites). One should have a rational approach to cases of ascites. Ask the following points.

- Whether it is associated with swelling of feet or face? If so where the swelling started? If swelling started in the feet before it appeared in the abdomen, the likely underlying cause is increased hydrostatic pressure, as seen in cardiac causes like right-sided heart failure, pericardial effusion, constrictive pericarditis, restrictive cardiomyo-pathy. In constrictive pericarditis, restrictive cardiomyopathy and in presence of tricuspid regurgitation and stenosis, ascites will be disproportionately more than the leg oedema. In fact, in constrictive pericarditis and restrictive cardiomyopathy, patient may complain of swelling of the abdomen before swelling of the feet. Swelling of the face precedes swelling of the abdomen in patients with nephrotic syndrome. If the patient categorically says that swelling of the abdomen started first and the swelling remained confined to the abdomen for a considerable time, the probable cause is in the abdomen itself, like tubercular peritonitis, malignant ascites, acute peritonitis. In cirrhosis of liver and in sub-acute hepatic failure (SAHF) though swelling of the abdomen develops earlier than swelling of the legs, but sooner or later leg oedema appears. In hepatic veno-occlusive disease there can be isolated ascites too.

- Whether it has occurred over a short duration (days) or over a long duration (months). Ascites develops over a short period in acute peritonitis; there can be acute increase in the size of ascites over existing long-standing ascites as seen in spontaneous bacterial peritonitis. Rapid accumulation of ascites can occur in malignant ascites and acute Budd-Chiari syndrome.

- Other associated symptoms should be asked for. Jaundice will suggest subacute hepatic failure and decompensated cirrhosis. GI bleeding can also occur in both these two conditions. Ascites with features of altered sensorium (encephalopathy) will suggest SAHF or cirrhosis of liver. Fever and abdominal pain occurs in acute peritonitis or spontaneous bacterial peritonitis, can be a feature of abdominal tuberculosis also. In most of the conditions of acute peritonitis the total clinical picture will give the clue to diagnosis. Dyspnoea antedates the development ascites in cases of congestive cardiac failure. Huge ascites alone can cause dyspnoea where it occurs late in the total clinical course. Marked weight loss with ascites may be of malignant or tubercular in origin. It also may be a part of malabsorption state (ascites due to hypoproteinemia).

VOMITING

Vomiting is a common symptom of many illnesses. It always does not mean that the disease is in the GI system. In evaluating a case presenting with vomiting the following points should be looked for.

Duration

Short Duration Vomiting

- Acute abdomen—invariably associated with abdominal pain
- Acute gastritis—May be due to **drugs** or **food poisoning**. So in all cases of vomiting of acute onset, ask for intake of drugs recently. Even some drugs administered parenterally can also cause vomiting like morphine and aminophylline. These latter drugs can cause vomiting by stimulating the CTZ/ vomiting center (so without causing gastritis). Unpalatable food or contaminated food can cause vomiting. It may be associated with diarrhoea

(enteritis). Other members who have taken the same food might be having similar complaints. Intake of **poisons** of various kinds also causes vomiting.

- Increased intracranial pressure—Meningitis, encephalitis, head injury, cerebrovascular accident, etc. can raise the intracranial pressure and can cause vomiting. So associated complaints like convulsion, fever, headache and altered sensorium should be enquired.
- Acute labyrinthitis—it will be associated with vertigo.
- Acute myocardial infarction particularly inferior wall—associated symptoms like chest pain, dyspnoea, etc. may be there.
- As a part of vasovagal syncope.
- Acute non-GI infections can also cause vomiting particularly in children.

Long Duration Vomiting

Vomiting may persist for several months. This may be again episodic or persistent.

Episodic vomiting—Encountered in some forms of epilepsy (autonomic), migraine (may or may not be associated with headache); Meniere's disease (will be associated with vertigo and impaired hearing). Motion sickness—occurs on movement in vehicles or merry-go-round games.

Persistent vomiting occurs in:
- Gastric outlet obstruction—Voluminous, projectile, vomitus containing food of previous days.
- Uraemia—may be associated with oliguria, swelling of the body, etc.

- Endocrinopathies—hypo- and hyperparathyroid states, Addison's disease
- Brain tumors—associated with localizing features and other features of raised intracranial tension.
- Gastric motility disorders—diabetic gastroparesis
- Morning sickness—in early pregnancy
- Psychogenic vomiting—there will not be true act of vomiting and usually does not lead to weight loss even if the complaint lasts for a long time.

Timing

- Morning—morning sickness of early pregnancy, water brush of APD, alcoholics
- Late afternoon—pyloric stenosis

Content of the Vomitus

- Always try to see yourself the content.
- Faeculent material—gastrocolic fistula
- Food of previous day—gastric outlet obstruction

Special Features

- Induced vomiting—Gastric ulcer
- Projectile vomiting—Raised intracranial pressure, pyloric stenosis, dynamic intestinal obstruction particularly if the obstruction is in the proximal intestine
- Motion induced—Motion sickness (usually in younger persons, more common in females)

Associated Symptoms

Out of all features the associated features help maximum to reach at a diagnosis. For instance:

Associated symptoms	Likely problem
Anorexia, nausea, oedema	... Uraemia
Anorexia, vomiting, weight loss	... Carcinoma stomach (prepyloric)
Diarrhoea	... Infective (food poisoning)
Abdominal pain and distention	... Intestinal obstruction
Fever, headache, altered sensorium	... Meningitis, encephalitis
Fever, jaundice	... Hepatitis, cholangitis
Sense of something moving in the abdomen	... Pyloric stenosis
Early pregnancy	... Morning sickness
Vertigo	... Labyrinthitis, Meniere's disease, acute cerebellar disease
Headache, convulsion, focal neurological deficit	... Intracranial space occupying lesion
Chest pain, dyspnoea, sweating	... Acute myocardial infarction
episodic headache	... Migraine
and so on.	

JAUNDICE

If a patient comes primarily with complaint of jaundice, it is imperative to decide whether it is haemolytic, hepatocellular or obstructive jaundice. This can be fairly confidently decided from the history.

Haemolytic

Often history dates back to childhood. It will be associated with growth retardation, bony changes, failure to thrive due to anaemia. In haemolytic conditions jaundice is usually mild, urine is not coloured. At times haemolytic jaundice can lead to obstructive jaundice (due to pigmentary gallstones), when it will behave like obstructive jaundice.

Hepatocellular

Common causes of hepatocellular jaundice are drug induced, viral and alcoholic. So enquire about intake of any hepatotoxic drug, alcoholism or prodromal symptoms of hepatitis (fever, anorexia, arthralgia, nausea, vomiting and malaise). Here the eyes will be yellow as well as the urine will be yellow.

Obstructive

In obstructive jaundice urine is coloured but stool is clay like. There may be pruritus and bleeding diathesis. It has to be remembered that cholestatic phase of hepatitis may have all these features.

If the patient concludes himself from the yellow colour of urine that he is suffering from jaundice, it may not be always true. Exclude history of intake of drugs which can cause yellow/orange coloured urine; like B complex vitamins, Rifampicin, Pyridium (Phenazopyridine). Excess intake of carrot can also cause yellowish urine. Less water intake can lead to passage of high coloured urine also.

Duration of jaundice can also help in the diagnosis of the probable cause of jaundice. Jaundice from childhood (may be of variable severity) suggests haemolytic jaundice or congenital hyperbilirubinaemia. Jaundice lasting for more than six months could be due to chronic hepatitis.

Pain in abdomen with jaundice is seen in hepatitis, obstruction due to gallstone and cholangitis. Painless progressive jaundice (obstructive nature) is likely to be due to carcinoma head of pancreas. Jaundice associated with mass in epigastric/ right hypochondrium may be due to carcinoma gallbladder, secondaries in the liver, distended gallbladder as in carcinoma head of pancreas. Jaundice with ascites will suggest subacute hepatic failure, decompensated cirrhosis, hepatic and peritoneal metastasis. Recurrent jaundice, fever, abdominal pain occurs in cholangitis. In addition to this, waxing and waning type of jaundice can be noticed in chronic hepatitis, haemolytic jaundice, periampullary carcinoma, obstruction of common bile duct due to a papilloma with peduncle.

GASTROINTESTINAL BLEEDING

Bleeding from the GI tract can manifest as haematemesis, melaena, haematochezia and bleeding per anum.

Haematemesis and Melaena

Haematemesis means vomiting of blood. Bleeding from stomach, duodenum and oesophagus (upper GI tract) will present like this. If the bleeding is small in amount, it may not cause blood vomiting, rather it will present as melaena. Melaena is commonly understood as black stool. But simple black stool may not be melaena. In true melaena stool will be black, tarry and will have offensive smell, with a tendency to stick to the lavatory pan. Black stool may be due to intake of iron, bismuth salts and charcoal. Whenever in doubt, try to see the stool yourself. When haematemesis and melaena both are present, there is little doubt.

In relation to haematemesis a few things need clarification, (1) Whether it is haematemesis or haemoptysis? (2) What is the amount? (3) What is the probable cause?

Whether it is haematemesis or haemoptysis?

In haematemesis there will be act of vomiting and nausea, whereas in haemoptysis there will be act of coughing. The blood in haemoptysis is frank red containing clot; in case of haematemesis blood will be coffee ground in colour (there may be small pieces of clots). Of course, massive haematemesis can be frank red and can contain clots. Vomitus may contain food material; there will be sputum or saliva (spurious haemoptysis) in case of haemoptysis. Haematemesis will be associated with melaena; haemoptysis usually does not. But if sufficient amount of blood is swallowed haemoptysis can also cause melaena. Bleeding from mouth should also be excluded in all cases; particularly if the amount of blood loss is small. If you get a chance to see the act of haematemesis/haemoptysis, it will be decisive.

What is the amount?

In relation to haematemesis often people exaggerate the amount of blood loss (discussed earlier). So in stead of frankly accepting the statements of the patient/ attendants objectively assess the amount of blood loss. From history it will not be easy to assess. However, if the patient has got excessive thirst, sweating, decreased urination, air hunger (restlessness) due to cerebral hypoxia, the blood loss is expected to be massive.

What is the probable cause?

From the history one can guess the probable cause of upper GI bleeding.

- Persistent vomiting and retching followed by haematemesis—Mallory-Weiss tear
- Known cirrhotic with massive haematemesis—Rupture oesophageal varices
- Marked anorexia/ new onset dyspepsia in a person above 40 years of age with weight loss with melaena/haematemesis—Carcinoma stomach
- Haematemesis followed by altered sensorium—Variceal bleeding precipitating hepatic encephalopathy
- Intake of NSAID followed by upper GI bleeding—Erosive gastritis
- Burn or other major physical illness with upper GI bleeding—Stress ulcer
- History suggestive of acid peptic disorder followed by upper GI bleeding—Peptic ulcer
- Upper GI bleeding with bleeding from other sites—Bleeding/coagulation disorder
- Repeated upper GI bleeding in young individuals without any deterioration of general health—Arterio venous malformation in the gastric wall

Haematochezia/ Bleeding per Anum

This means passage of altered blood per anum, at times it is also used synonymously as bleeding per anum. Altered blood means it is neither fresh blood nor tarry blood as in melaena. But from the patient's point of view it may not be possible to distinguish bleeding per anum and passage of altered blood. True bleeding per anum means passage of frank blood which may be complained as passage of blood in drops or jets or streaking of blood on the surface of stool. This blood if stays on the pan for some time will clot. This is seen in ano-rectal pathology like piles, fissures, rectal carcinoma, and rectal polyp. Piles is usually painless unless complicated (thrombosis or infected), bleeding often follows passage of stool in drops or jets; complaint is often there for a long time. Recent constipation with frank bleeding per anum suggests carcinoma rectum. Blood streaking on the surface of formed stool and associated with painful defaecation is indicative of fissure. In case of a child with bleeding per anum it is usually rectal polyp. In cases of bleeding per anum it is required to exclude bacillary/amoebic dysentery. I have seen cases of bleeding piles being treated as bacillary dysentery and vice versa. A detail history and visual inspection of the stool will be decisive in most cases unless both the conditions coexist.

Altered stool occurs if the bleeding is from below the ligament of Treitz and above rectum. Some of the causes of haematochezia are bleeding in enteric fever, bleeding from intestinal polyps, mesenteric artery occlusion, bleeding from Meckel's diverticulum, carcinoma colon, ulcerative colitis and so on. It can also occur in association with upper GI bleeding with hurried intestinal transit.

DYSPHAGIA

Dysphagia means difficulty in swallowing food/drink. Patient may complain differently like he may tell that he feels the sensation of sticking of food while swallowing, he may say he feels the sensation of a lump in the throat though there is no true difficulty in swallowing. The latter is not true dysphagia. One should not confuse dysphagia with refusal to take food which is seen in rabies, tetanus and hysterical conditions. In conditions of odynophagia (painful deglutition) there can be refusal to take food also. Whenever dealing with a case of dysphagia a few points are to be clarified. These are:

- Whether it is mechanical dysphagia (the lumen of the oesophagus is narrowed) or it is motor dysphagia (coordinated contraction of the oesophageal muscles is not there)?
- Is it painful (odynophagia)?
- It is at which phase of deglutition?
- What are the associated complaints?
- How it has started?

In mechanical dysphagia there occurs dysphagia to solid foods initially, which may be helped by a draught of water, but in the late stage there will be dysphagia to liquids as well. In motor dysphagia there is dysphagia to liquid and solid from the beginning. A typical pattern of dysphagia is seen in scleroderma. Here the patient complains of dysphagia to solid in all postures whereas there will be dysphagia to liquid only in recumbent posture, not in upright posture. Some of the common causes of mechanical dysphagia are carcinoma, stricture, compression from outside (as in lymphoma, bronchogenic carcinoma and aortic aneurysm, etc). Some common causes of motor dysphagia are achalasia, scleroderma, and diffuse spasm of the oesophagus, Chagas' disease, and motor neurone disease.

Painful dysphagia occurs in peritonsillar/ tonsillar abscess, retropharyngeal abscess; can also be seen in oesophageal candidiasis.

Dysphagia occurring in the initial phase of deglutition (oropharyngeal) may be due to mechanical cause, but more frequently it is of neurogenic in origin. There is non-contraction/uncoordinated contraction of the pharyngeal muscles, upper oesophageal sphincter or of the striated muscles in the upper oesophagus, which may be due to nuclear or infranuclear involvement of the vagus nerve (with or without ninth nerve). Involvement of bilateral corticobulbar fibers can cause dysphagia (pseudobulbar palsy), but unilateral lesion does not cause any problem. Here there will be associated complaints like dysarthria and dysphonia. Nasal regurgitation of food/ drink, induction of cough on deglutition occurs mostly in lower motor neurone type of bulbar palsy. If a patient does not have dysphagia/ dysphonia/ dysarthria but attempt to swallow induces cough, think of the possibility of tracheo-oesophageal fistula.

Dysphagia in other parts of the oesophagus is more often mechanical. Often the patient is able to locate the site of dysphagia which is more or less correct.

Onset and course of dysphagia also helps in reaching at the diagnosis.

- Abrupt onset of dysphagia occurs in bolus impaction or impaction of foreign body. Can also be seen in bulbar palsy and following ingestion of corrosive agents.
- Progressive dysphagia of weeks to months' duration suggests carcinoma.
- Transient dysphagia occurs in inflammatory conditions.
- Long-standing dysphagia of several months to years' duration can occur in stricture, oesophageal ring and motor dysphagia.

Past History in a Case of Dysphagia

History of radiation, intake of corrosive agents, acid reflux suggest stricture.

DIARRHOEA AND CONSTIPATION

Before collecting details of the history of diarrhoea or constipation, one should enquire about the usual bowel habit of the individual because normal bowel habit varies widely.

Diarrhoea

In case of diarrhoea the following aspects should be enquired:
a. Duration
b. Frequency
c. Volume of stool
d. Colour and odour
e. Associated complaints

Diarrhoea of Short Duration (less than 2 weeks)

Mostly here the cause is infective in origin; but may be due to intake of toxic substances or drugs. If there is history of intake of contaminated foods or drinks, infective cause is suggested. Many people might be suffering from similar illness (epidemic/miniepidemic). Always take history of intake of any drugs. Many antibiotics (amoxicillin, ampicillin, tetracycline, cephalosporins) can cause diarrhoea. If diarrhoea is associated with fever, it goes in favour of infective diarrhoea. Diarrhoea with vomiting suggests toxin-mediated diarrhoea; may be bacterial toxins also. In toxigenic diarrhoea there is either no abdominal pain or slight abdominal pain. In *entero invasive* diarrhoea there can be fever and abdominal pain. Passage of blood or mucus suggests invasive diarrhoea. But even in invasive diarrhoea there can be watery diarrhoea at the beginning. Passage of little amount of stool with blood and mucus several times a day (may be > 10 times) associated with tenesmus (painful straining for defaecation with passage of small amount of stool) suggests bacillary dysentery. Fishy odour of stool will be there in amoebic dysentery. Melaena and bloody diarrhoea has been already discussed. Always try to see the stool yourself in doubtful situations.

Diarrhoea of Long Duration (Chronic Diarrhoea)

When diarrhoea lasts for more than two weeks, it is chronic diarrhoea. This may be persistent or intermittent. The causes of such diarrhoea are inflammatory, osmotic, secretory or intestinal dysmotility.

Inflammatory: The conditions are regional ileitis, ulcerative colitis and intestinal tuberculosis. There will be passage of blood, mucus and/or pus. Constitutional symptoms of fever, arthralgia/ arthritis, weight loss may be associated. Features of subacute intestinal obstruction (intermittent abdominal pain, vomiting) may be present in intestinal tuberculosis and Crohn's disease. Intestinal tuberculosis may be associated with tuberculous ascites. Due to protein losing enteropathy there can be peripheral oedema in all these conditions. Carcinoma of the proximal colon can cause diarrhoea and weight loss though it is not an inflammatory condition.

Osmotic diarrhoea: This is mostly due to maldigestion (due to exocrine pancreatic insufficiency) or malabsorption. There is no blood or mucus in the stool. Volume of stool is large, floats on water and sticks to the lavatory pan (steatorrhoea). Weight loss is invariably present. Ask for any specific food intolerance like milk (Lactose intolerance) or wheat products (Gluten enteropathy).

Secretory diarrhoea: Passage of watery stool episodically or chronically can be due to secretion of a lot of fluids into the GI tract under influence of certain GI hormones like Gastrin (Zollinger-Ellison syndrome), vasoactive intestinal peptide (pancreatic cholera), and serotonin (carcinoid syndrome).

Some other causes are villous adenoma of the rectum where there is diarrhoea due to increased secretion also. In medullary carcinoma of thyroid there can be chronic diarrhoea also.

Intestinal dysmotility: The causes are thyrotoxicosis, irritable bowel syndrome (IBS), and long standing diabetes mellitus. In IBS there is no weight loss, no nocturnal diarrhoea and there can be alternate diarrhoea and constipation. In thyrotoxicosis other features will be obvious. In diabetes other features of autonomic neuropathy may be present.

Spurious diarrhoea: Passage of small amount of formed stool frequently can be due to incomplete evacuation. This is seen in growth in distal colon leading to faecal impaction above.

CONSTIPATION

Though constipation is a common problem but rarely it is the chief complaint. Often other symptoms are more troublesome which draws the attention of the patient. If at all at any time, the patient presents with constipation as the primary complaint, the most important point to be collected is duration.

If it is from very early childhood (newborn stage) and it is marked, it could be Hirschsprung's disease. Excluding Hirschsprung's disease other causes of prolonged constipation are idiopathic, hypothyroid state, Parkinson's disease, Dementic states, other paralytic states like paraplegia, Chagas' disease, IBS. In IBS there can be alternate diarrhoea with constipation. If the constipation is of short duration, ask for any recent change in food habit or intake of drugs. Intake of food rich in animal protein can cause constipation. Several drugs can cause constipation like antipsychotic drugs, iron, calcium, codeine and other opium alkaloids, calcium channel antagonists and others. Distal colonic obstruction can also present with recent onset constipation. In anal fissure and in thrombosed piles there is pain during defaecation so that the patient is afraid of passing stool which leads to constipation. Obstipation (no passage of flatus or faeces) occurs in intestinal obstruction.

WEIGHT LOSS

Weight loss is a common complaint in comparison to weight gain. However, the amount of weight loss is often exaggerated. One has to be certain that, there is true weight loss. This has been already discussed. Once it is established that there is weight loss it should be viewed seriously because invariably it is due to organic diseases, some of them may be grave conditions. Though it is being discussed in GI system, it does not always mean that the underlying condition is in the GI system. In most of the situations the cause is obvious from the associated symptoms. Some of the common causes and their associated symptoms are as follows.

1. Polyuria, polyphagia, polydipsia—IDDM (Type I diabetes mellitus)

2. Inability to take food (dysphagia)—Carcinoma oesophagus/stricture oesophagus

3. Not getting enough food—Malnutrition. More common in children, but can be seen in adult as well

4. Inability to retain food (prolonged vomiting)—Gastric outlet obstruction

5. Exophthalmos, goitre, increased appetite, excessive sweating—Thyrotoxicosis

6. Prolonged fever, persistent cough, haemoptysis, etc—Tuberculosis

7. Voluminous stool, foul smelling, sticky stool—Malabsorption state

8. All malignancies are associated with significant weight loss and most of them will be obvious from the other symptoms. But always the primary may not be obvious. In such situations the cause may lie in the GI system (stomach, colon, and pancreas) and in female it could be in the uterus.

9. AIDS—It is invariably associated with weight loss. Associated symptoms like prolonged fever, prolonged diarrhoea, and generalized lymphadenopathy with history of multiple sexual exposures will suggest the diagnosis.

10. Cirrhosis of liver—Upper part of the body is emaciated; lower part is bloated due to oedema and ascites.

A few more conditions can cause weight loss but the cause may not be too obvious, though meticulously taken history will reveal important clues to diagnosis. These are Addison's disease, panhypopituitarism, overdieting, anorexia nervosa, chronic infective conditions like subacute bacterial endocarditis and amoebic liver abscess.

History in Genitourinary Disorders

> *Before putting any hollow thing (like a needle) into the body, look for its patency.*

Patient with urinary problem may present with the following complaints as single or in combinations.

- Oliguria
- Polyuria
- Frequency of urination
- Pain
- Haematuria
- Swelling of the body
- Retention of urine
- Hesitancy, urgency, incontinence
- Fever
- Lump

OLIGURIA

When the urine output is less than 500 ml in twenty-four hours it is called oliguria. This amount of urine output is required to wash out the daily nitrogenous waste products. This has to be objectively established by asking the patient to measure the 24-hour urinary output. Once it is established, enquire about the duration of complaint.

Oliguria of Short Duration

If the patient has developed oliguria over a short duration (within days), it suggests acute renal failure. This may be due to prerenal conditions like hypovolemia as seen in diarrhoea, vomiting, acute massive blood loss, burns, etc. It may be due to renal conditions like acute glomerulonephritis (AGN), involvement of the kidney due to other diseases like complicated malaria, snake bite, intravascular haemolysis, urate nephropathy, myeloma protein nephropathy (light chain), myoglobin precipitation in the tubules as in rhabdomyolysis and so on. If oliguria lasts for a few days and the patient continues to take water as usual, oedema will develop. Oliguria due to AGN will be accompanied by haematuria. In angioneurotic oedema a similar picture like AGN develops but here swelling of the body develops early, oliguria if at all develops will be later than swelling of the body (reverse of AGN). There will be no haematuria. In both there can be dyspnoea, but if there is stridor (due to laryngeal oedema) it goes more in favour of angioneurotic oedema.

Oliguria of Long Duration

If the patient complains of oliguria of longer duration (weeks to months), invariably it will be associated with oedema. Oliguria lasting for more than two weeks and less than three months will suggest RPGN (Rapidly progressive glomerulo-nephritis); and if the duration of oliguria lasts for more than three months, it is suggestive of chronic renal failure. This differentiation may not be possible from history only, it needs investigation.

ANURIA

There will be no urination in twenty-four hours. True anuria is extremely uncommon in medical situations. It is usually due to obstructive uropathy; either the obstruction is at the bladder neck or accidental ligation of both ureters during surgery. Bilateral obstruction of ureter leading to anuria is at times possible in retroperitoneal fibrosis. Bilateral occlusion of renal vessels (both arteries/both veins) can also cause anuria, which is equally uncommon. Hence, it can be concluded that in all cases of anuria urinary tract obstruction must be excluded. If the obstruction is below the bladder neck, there will be fullness of the bladder which is quite painful if the sensory system is intact (above S2, S3). Even an unconscious patient becomes restless due to full bladder. It is easy to detect by inspection and percussion. The obstruction to the bladder neck need not be structural always; it may be physiological also, due to impairment of neurogenic control (lesion in the spinal cord or cauda equina). However, unilateral lesion may not cause retention of urine; if at all for a transient period. Retention of urine due to neurological cause is easy to diagnose except in a few situations like intramedullary lesions in the early stage.

POLYURIA/ NOCTURIA

When the twenty-four-hour urinary output is more than three liters it is said to be polyuria. Like oliguria, this has to be objectively assessed. Ask the patient to collect urine for 24 hours for a few days and confirm that there is polyuria. Once it is established one should try to find out a cause. Some of the common causes of polyuria are diabetes mellitus, diuretic therapy, polyuric phase of acute renal failure, diabetes insipidus, some forms of chronic renal failure, compulsive water drinking (psychogenic polydipsia) and a few more. So in the history collect the following data.

Associated with polyphagia, polydipsia, susceptibility to infections and others—diabetes mellitus.

History of intake of diuretics, patient may not be able to name the drugs; hence, check the drugs/prescription physically.

Preceding history of oliguria—polyuric phase of acute renal failure.

Long-standing history of anorexia, nausea, vomiting and swelling of the body—chronic renal failure

It is not possible to come to a conclusion from history about compulsive water drinking and diabetes insipidus. Even with detail investigations it may not be possible to differentiate these two conditions.

Nocturia is nothing but nocturnal polyuria. In the initial stages of all causes of polyuria patient feels that he has to get up more frequently at night to pass urine. Truly there is polyuria both at night as well as at daytime; but as the patient has to get up from sleep frequently to pass urine, he appreciates that urination is more frequent at night. Nobody counts how many times one passes urine at daytime. There can be nocturia in conditions of frequency also and in bladder neck obstruction due to benign hypertrophy of prostate.

FREQUENCY OF URINATION

Frequency of urination is nothing but passage of urine at frequent intervals. This may be associated with increased volume of urination when it becomes polyuria (discussed earlier). In true frequency there will be passage of small amount of urine at a time. There are several conditions where this can occur, but the primary mechanism is an irritable bladder which senses to be full even at a lesser volume. This is commonly due to inflammation of the bladder wall as in cystitis, but can also be due to neurologic instability (particularly increased tone of the trigone of the bladder under influence of sympathetic nerves as happens just before examination/ interview). Frequency of urination may be due to true reduction of the capacity of the bladder. This may be due to inability to distend as seen in infiltration of the bladder wall (malignant/ tubercular) or growth inside the bladder lumen.

PAIN

Various types of pain are possible in diseases of the urinary system.

* Fixed pain in the flanks occurs in perinephric abscess and acute pyelonephritis. In these conditions pain is severe and is associated with high fever. Constant aching type of pain in the renal angle is possible in obstruction at pelvi ureteric junction.
* Colicky pain can be felt in ureteric obstruction. Typically in ureteric colic pain starts in the loin and radiates to the groin inner side of thigh, and to the genitals. The quality of pain is like other types of colicky pain (described in GI system).
* Dysuria—A type of discomfort felt during passage of urine (often burning type) is felt in inflammation of lower urinary tract. In inflammation of urinary bladder maximum pain will be towards the end of urination, and in urethral inflammation maximum discomfort is during the flow of urine or at the beginning.
* Dull aching suprapubic pain is felt when the bladder is full, also in cystitis.
* Pain in the perineum or in the rectum may be due to prostatitis or prostatic abscess.

FEVER

Fever in urinary disorders usually means infection. However, fever can be due to renal tumors also; particularly hypernephroma. Urinary tract infection is traditionally classified into upper urinary tract infection and lower urinary tract infection (bladder and urethra). In upper urinary tract infection (pyelonephritis) fever is high, associated with chill and rigor and there will be pain in the renal angle. It has to be remembered that in chronic pyelonephritis there may not be fever at all. In lower urinary tract infection fever is usually low to moderate grade, associated with dysuria, urgency, and dull suprapubic pain. Prostatic abscess and prostatitis can present as pyrexia of unknown origin. In prostatic abscess there will be pain in the perineum.

HAEMATURIA

In haematuria patient complains of passage of red coloured urine. The colour of urine varies, depending on the amount of blood present. It may be smoky if the amount of blood is small and it may be frankly red if the blood amount is more. Even there can be haematuria without change of colour of the urine as in infective endocarditis (microscopic haematuria). All red urine need not be haematuria. It can be due to haemoglobinuria also. Differentiation of these two conditions depends on the chemical and microscopic examination of the urine. In haemoglobinuria chemical test for blood will be positive and RBC in urine will be absent. Hemoglobinuria suggests intravascular haemolysis. Ask the patient in which phase of urination he notices haematuria. If it is in the initial phase, the cause is likely to be in the urethra. If it is in the terminal phase, the likely cause is to be in the urinary bladder; and if the haematuria is uniformly throughout the act of urination (total), the likely site of bleeding is in the kidney or ureter. If the patient is not able to tell, he can be asked to collect urine in three clear bottles from initial, middle and terminal phase of urination and you can see yourself. In a case of haematuria a few more points can help the diagnosis. These are—geographical area, history of trauma, duration, associated complaint.

Geographical Area

In a tropical country like India, Filaria is a common cause, in Egypt it may be due to Schistosoma haematobium infestation.

History of Trauma

Direct or indirect trauma to the kidney or urinary tract can cause haematuria. Trauma may be road traffic accident, fall from a height or blunt injury to abdomen. Trauma to urinary tract may be due to catheterization or instrumentation. Perineal injury can lead to urethral rupture (at times the trauma may appear to be trivial).

Associated Complaint

It is the associated complaint which gives maximum clue to the diagnosis.

a. If there is bleeding from other sites, it could be a bleeding disorder like thrombocytopenia (as in idiopathic thrombocytopenic purpura), hypoplastic anaemia or acute leukaemia. It may be a coagulation disorder also; particularly excess of anticoagulants.

b. Fever: If the fever is of short duration, it may be cystitis; if fever is of long duration, it may be infective endocarditis, hypernephroma, renal tuberculosis.

c. Feeling of a lump: Hypernephroma and other kidney tumors like Wilms' tumor, polycystic kidney disease. Unlike hypernephroma, haematuria is late in Wilms' tumor.

d. Pain: Pain will be present in trauma, stone in the renal pelvis or in the ureter. Passage of a clot through the ureter (bleeding due to other causes) can also cause colicky pain.

e. Swelling of the body: If haematuria is associated with swelling of the body, it could be acute glomerulonephritis (AGN) or some specific histological varieties of nephrotic syndrome. Both can also be distinguished from history. In AGN there will be oliguria and the total duration of complaints will be short; whereas in nephrotic syndrome urine output is usually normal and the duration of complaints is longer.

f. Chyluria: If haematuria is associated with chyluria, there are only a very few causes like Bancroftian filariasis, tuberculosis and lymphoma.

g. Haemoptysis: If haematuria is associated with haemoptysis, it could be Goodpasture's syndrome or renal tuberculosis with pulmonary tuberculosis.

h. Weight loss: Can be found in renal cell carcinoma or renal tuberculosis; can also be seen in malignant bladder tumors also.

Painless, profuse and paroxysmal haematuria is seen in papilloma of the bladder. Painless recurrent haematuria can also occur in IgA nephropathy and thin basement membrane disease.

PASSAGE OF WHITISH URINE

If a patient complains of passage of whitish urine, it could be due to pus, excess of phosphates in the urine or chyle. Frank pus discharge per urethra can occur in gonococcal urethritis; whereas passage of turbid urine commonly suggests lower urinary tract infection. Passage of whitish urine may be due to phosphaturia where particulate materials can be seen in the urine, particularly in a long-standing catheterized patient. In chyluria urine is white. Fat globules can be seen to be floating on the surface of the urine. This has been discussed earlier.

LUMP

At times patient may come with complain of feeling of a mass in the abdomen. The mass is invariably due to a kidney mass or due to a full bladder (see retention). By the time kidney is felt as a mass it is quite big. It may be due to renal tumors, polycystic kidney disease or hydronephrosis. Renal mass in childhood could be due to Wilms' tumor.

RETENTION/HESITANCY

Retention of urine (Full bladder) is easy to detect as it is painful unless patient has got loss of sensation above S2 and S3. Often he will be complaining of difficulty in passing urine or no passage of urine; the mass will be a suprapubic mass. Some common causes of retention of urine are congenital posterior urethral valve, phimosis, benign hyperplasia of prostate, carcinoma prostate, stricture urethra and stone or tumor at bladder neck or below. All these are primarily surgical conditions. Common medical cause of retention of urine is interruption of nerve supply to the bladder (bilateral). Before the patient develops retention of urine he may appreciate difficulty in initiation of urination or there may be dribbling of urine. Patient may take longer time to complete the act of urination. This is applicable both for neurological as well as for surgical causes. Retention of urine in female due to surgical causes is relatively uncommon. However, some conditions peculiar to females can cause retention like carcinoma cervix, big cervical polyp, retroverted gravid uterus.

INCONTINENCE

This is the reverse of retention. Here the patient is not able to hold urine so that he passes urine in his cloth. The basic problem is lack of tone in the bladder neck (internal and external sphincter of the bladder). Lesion is in the inhibitory pathway; may be in the spinal cord, conus medullaris or cauda equina. There are several types of incontinence like true incontinence, overflow incontinence and stress incontinence. Most often it is neurological in origin, but stress incontinence particularly in female may be there without any neurological lesion; usually it is seen following childbirth and in uterine prolapse. In male it can follow bladder neck surgery. True incontinence may be due to injury to external sphincter or may be due to urinary fistula.

SWELLING OF THE BODY

If a patient comes with complaints of swelling of the body, it may be a cardiovascular problem (discussed earlier), kidney problem, liver disease (discussed earlier), diseases of the GI system (protein losing enteropathy) and a few other situations where there is increased capillary permeability like angioneurotic oedema, wet beriberi, epidemic dropsy. So whenever there is swelling of the body, exclude kidney disease. Kidney diseases causing oedema are acute glumerulonephritis (AGN), nephrotic syndrome, acute renal failure (ARF), chronic renal failure (CRF) and RPGN (rapidly progressive glumerulonephritis). In AGN and nephrotic syndrome swelling may appear first in the lower eyelid. In all except nephrotic syndrome and some forms of CRF there will be oliguria. Duration of oliguria may help to differentiate ARF, RPGN and CRF. Other associated symptoms may also help.

SIGNIFICANT PAST HISTORY IN URINARY DISEASES

In a case with urinary disease several past histories may be significant depending on the situation. Some of the examples are given herewith.

- Hypertension—In a case of CRF.
- Tuberculosis—In a case of genitourinary tuberculosis
- Recurrent urinary tract infection—In CRF
- Sickle cell disease—Nephrotic syndrome
- Skin infection—Acute glomerulonephritis
- Diabetes mellitus—Nephrotic syndrome, CRF
- Collagen diseases—Nephrotic syndrome, CRF
- Gonococcal urethritis—Stricture urethra
- Perineal injury—Stricture urethra
- Exposure to nephrotoxic drugs—ARF, CRF

- Hypovolemic conditions (diarrhoea, vomiting, burn, massive blood loss)—ARF

And so on.

Family History

Though it is not very important in diseases of the urinary system, it may be important in a few conditions like polycystic kidney disease and Alport's syndrome, hereditary tubular disorders like medullary cystic kidney, medullary sponge kidney, congenital nephrogenic diabetes insipidus and others.

Personal History

It is not very important in most cases of urinary disorders.

14

History in Unconscious Patients

> *Plan, prioritize and know the cost effectiveness before subjecting any case for investigation.*

It is my observation over the years that most of the students get confused when they deal with an unconscious patient. Any unconscious patient is a critically ill patient. Approach to these cases must be clear, quick and rational. Like other systemic illnesses, the key point lies in the history taking and meticulous examinations. Failing to do this may lead to a lot of unnecessary investigations and wastage of valuable time, which may at times cost the life of the patient.

The common causes of unconsciousness are as follows:

A. Head injury
B. Cerebrovascular disorders
  - Cerebral haemorrhage
  - Cerebral thrombosis
  - Cerebral embolism
  - Hypertensive encephalopathy
  - Subarachnoid haemorrhage

C. Infective conditions affecting the brain
- Encephalitis
- Meningitis
- Cerebral malaria
- Typhoid encephalopathy
- Brain abscess

D. Metabolic
- Uraemic encephalopathy
- Hepatic encephalopathy
- Anoxic encephalopathy
  - Hanging and drowning
- Carbon dioxide narcosis
- Electrolyte imbalance
  - Hyponatraemia
  - Hypercalcaemia
- Coma in Diabetes
  - Hypoglycaemia
  - Diabetic ketoacidosis
  - Hyperosmolar

E. Intoxication
- Alcohol (Ethyl and Methyl)
- Barbiturate
- Opium alkaloids
- Benzodiazepines
- Other antipsychotic drugs
- Anti-diabetic drugs
- Organophosphorus compounds and others

Majority of the cases will fall under these categories.
However, there are some uncommon causes like myxoedema

coma, pituitary haemorrhage, advanced diffuse cerebral atherosclerosis, hyperviscosity states, etc.

From Whom History to be Collected?

Because these patients are not able to narrate their history, if at all not reliable; history should be collected from a person who was actually present at the time of occurrence of the illness. He may be the spouse, father, mother, servant, school teacher, colleague, class mate, room mate and so on. If the incident occurred on the road, the person who attended him first should give the history.

Exclude Head Injury

The causes enumerated here are mostly medical causes except head injury. Hence, while dealing with an unconscious patient first exclude head injury. It is simple on most of the occasions. Because there will be history of direct injury to head and following which the patient lost consciousness. But at times the trauma may be less obvious, because it may be an indirect injury, for example, a fall. Here it is required to know whether the fall is first (head injury) or the unconsciousness is first (stroke). This can be established fairly well if the circumstances under which fall occurred can be known.

Where the patient fell? Whether the place was dark or lighted? Was there anything to stumble over? Was the place slippery (as a bathroom)? A person will not ordinarily fall in a known place even in darkness unless the place is slippery or there is something to stumble over. The size of the object over which the patient stumbled over should be sufficiently large or heavy to make him fall; so enquire about it. The patient might have missed a step in a staircase and fall which is possible in darkness. Considering these entire points one should be able to decide that there was sufficient reason for fall; so that fall is first and the unconsciousness is the effect. So it could be head injury. Other points which may help are if there is sufficiently large swelling over scalp, if there is bleeding from the nostril or from external auditory meatus it could be head injury.

After head injury is excluded look for the following points to reach at a provisional diagnosis.

Was the Patient Absolutely Normal before it Happened?

An apparently normal person may become unconscious in cerebrovascular disorders or due to consumption of poisons. The hallmark of a cerebrovascular disorder is a focal neurological deficit which can be better known by examining the patient, but can be known if the attendants are able to tell that the patient is not moving a particular limb/limbs. This can also be noted by closely observing the patient (whether any particular limb the patient is moving or not, position of the limbs, position and movement of eyes) while history is being collected. However, there may not be focal neurological deficit in hypertensive encephalopathy and subarachnoid haemorrhage.

In case of consumption of poison ask the attendants to search for open strips of tablets or bottles in the vicinity of occurrence of the incident. These things might be left in the room or might have been thrown out of the window. I remember a medical student who attempted to commit suicide who had hidden the open stripes of tablets underneath her mattress (she consumed glibenclamide and propranolol together). There might be smell of the particular poison from the breath of the patient as in alcohol and organophosphorus compounds. If intake of certain drugs is suspected, enquire if any of the family members is taking some drugs for a long time like antidiabetic drugs, antiepileptic drugs or any other. I remember a case where the elder child had accidentally consumed all the iron tablets of the mother who was taking them for her continuing second pregnancy. This type of enquiry not only helps to know the drug (poison) but the amount of it (by deducting the number of remaining tablets from those supposed to be present by that particular day). I also remember a lady student who consumed phenobarbiturate tablets getting from her room mate who was taking for epilepsy.

What was the Starting Complaint?

Fever

Ask for history of fever before the onset of unconsciousness. If the starting complaint is fever, it is likely to be an infective condition affecting the brain like encephalitis, meningitis, cerebral malaria, typhoid encephalopathy. Encephalopathy due to typhoid occurs after two to three weeks of continued fever. If the fever is associated with skin rash, it could be viral meningoencephalitis and meningococcal septicemia. It has to be remembered that fever can occur in other conditions like intracerebral haemorrhage/ subarachnoid haemorrhage, but in these conditions fever is not the starting complaint, fever occurs later.

Convulsion

If the disease started with convulsion, it could be post-ictal state. Following repeated convulsion patient remains unconscious for some time. Hence, the patient might be a known case of epilepsy (either inadequately treated or discontinued treatment). In a pregnant woman similar thing can happen in eclampsia which is not difficult to diagnose if blood pressure is recorded. This should be remembered that convulsion can occur in almost all the causes of unconsciousness mentioned above, but rarely in these conditions it is the starting complaint.

Jaundice

If the patient had jaundice before becoming unconscious, it could be hepatic encephalopathy. If this is due to cirrhosis, history suggestive of cirrhosis will be obtained (ascites and leg oedema of long duration, haematemesis); and if this is due to hepatitis, there will be jaundice of short duration, and if at all there will be oedema or ascites, it will be of short duration (subacute hepatic failure). Jaundice in an unconscious patient may be found in complicated malaria and leptospirosis; but in these conditions rarely, it is the starting complaint, often other features dominate the total clinical picture.

Headache

Headache might be the starting complaint in subarachnoid haemorrhage or intracerebral haemorrhage; but headache is the outstanding complaint (often it is bursting type) of subarachnoid haemorrhage. Headache may be there in meningitis and encephalitis also but in these conditions fever occurs earlier or together. In subarachnoid haemorrhage fever may occur later on, never the starting complaint.

Under what Circumstances it Happened?

An otherwise normal person becoming unconscious following exposure to hot weather (working/walking under hot sun) could be a heat stroke; often the body temperature of these patients is very high. Similarly, prolonged exposure to too cold environment may cause hypothermia; so the body temperature will be too less.

A person recovered unconscious from a burning house is likely to be suffering from carbon monoxide (CO) poisoning. Similarly, CO poisoning can occur in persons sleeping in a closed room with generator on.

Two other forms of anoxic encephalopathy commonly encountered are hanging and drowning. In these situations diagnosis is obvious.

Was the Patient Receiving any Drug before the Onset?

Look for the drugs the patient might be taking before becoming unconscious. Not only see the prescription, verify them physically too. Some drugs might be still there in the pocket of the patient. These drugs themselves might be the cause of unconsciousness or the underlying illness for which the drugs were taken might be the cause. Also, verify if the drugs have been taken as per the prescription or in excess. The drugs might have been dispensed wrongly by the chemist (so physical verification of the drug is important). There are several such examples. I remember a case, where it was prescribed to take DIMOL but the drug served was DAONIL which the patient took and landed up in hypoglycemic coma.

A patient receiving diuretics for other illnesses may develop confusional state due to hyponatraemia.

Is there any other Specific Associated Symptoms?

Hyperventilation: If the patient is taking deep and rapid respiration, it could be uraemic, diabetic ketoacidotic, hyperosmolar coma or other forms of acidosis. Neurogenic hyperventilation is also possible in situations with raised intracranial pressure.

Excessive sweating: This may be due to hypoglycaemia or in cases where fever has just subsided in a febrile patient.

Polyuria: It could be symptom of uncontrolled diabetes mellitus and in some cases of chronic renal failure. In polyuric phase of acute renal failure patient may develop hypo-natraemic encephalopathy.

Oliguria: Irrespective of any cause if the patient has not received sufficient water there will be decreased urination. Hence, before considering oliguria as a complaint patient's hydration status must be assessed. In spite of the hydration status being good if the patient is oliguric it could be a case of uraemic encephalopathy (may be ARF, RPGN or CRF).

Swelling of the body: Loss of consciousness with swelling of the body is possible in chronic liver disease (hepatic encephalopathy), or kidney disease (Uraemic encephalopathy).

Bleeding from other sites: Bleeding from other sites may be due to a bleeding disorder which itself might have caused intracerebral bleed. This may be due to leptospirosis as well. Only upper gastrointestinal bleeding is not very important because it can occur in several conditions due to stress ulceration.

History of Past Illnesses

Hypertension: Look for the documentary evidences of hypertension. Whether he was taking the drugs regularly or discontinued before the onset of the illness (which is fairly common). A patient of uncontrolled hypertension may suffer from hypertension-related conditions like cerebrovascular accident (haemorrhage, thrombosis, subarachnoid haemorrhage) or hypertensive encephalopathy.

Diabetes mellitus: If the patient was a known case of diabetes mellitus, ask for the documentary evidence for it and verify whether he was continuing the drugs regularly or not, whether hyperglycemia was well controlled or not. Discontinuation of the drugs may cause diabetic ketoacidosis or hyperosmolar coma. Was his diet habit regular, particularly on the day of occurrence? Hypoglycemic coma occurs under certain situations; like taking the anti-diabetic drugs and missing a meal or taking less food or wrongly taking excess of the drugs or vomiting soon after intake of food. One should be sure that diagnosis of diabetes mellitus is reliable. I have seen cases being prescribed anti-diabetic drugs on detection of reducing substances in urine (Benedict's test) and patients presenting with hypoglycaemic coma.

COPD: If the patient was suffering from COPD (chronic obstructive pulmonary disease) he might develop confusional state due to excess of carbon dioxide (CO_2 narcosis).

Hypothyroid state: History of hypothyroidism may be obtained from the patient. If so, how long the thyroxin has been discontinued? Myxoedema coma occurs in patients of long-standing hypothyroid state, by which time the very appearance of the patient may be suggestive of the diagnosis.

Chronic kidney disease: Any form of long-standing kidney disease can cause chronic renal failure leading to uraemic encephalopathy.

Unconsciousness due to hypercalcaemia and hyper-viscosity is rare and often the underlying cause is more obvious.

History in Patients with Transient Loss of Unconsciousness

At times people present with transient loss of consciousness. Some common causes of such problems are transient ischaemic attacks involving the vertebrobasilar territory, syncope of different aetiologies and Stokes-Adams attacks and epileptic attacks.

By far the commonest cause is syncope and the commonest form of syncope is vasovagal syncope. The circumstances under which syncope develops will be decisive to know. For example: hearing a bad news, seeing a frightening scene, prolonged standing under the sun all can lead to syncope. Nausea is a frequent accompanying symptom of vasovagal syncope. The other type of syncope is micturition syncope which has a tendency to occur repeatedly and each time during micturition, often micturating in erect posture. Syncope of cardiac origin is either arrhythmic or due to left ventricular outflow tract obstruction. If it is due to arrhythmia [(Ventricular tachyarrhythmia or marked bradycardia of any cause (sick sinus syndrome, complete heart block)], it can occur in any posture. Remember that vasovagal syncope occurs in upright posture. In case of syncope recovery is quick and often complete. Rarely it may be associated with convulsion.

In case of transient ischaemic attacks of vertebrobasilar territory, there will be premonitory symptoms like vertigo, diplopia and unsteadiness of gait before loss of consciousness. Even these symptoms may persist for some time after the patient regains consciousness.

In case of epilepsy recovery is often late and incomplete. Following recovery patient may remain in an amnesic state for some time, may feel undue tiredness and there could be transient focal neurological deficit (Todd's palsy). History of tongue bite and involuntary passage of urine will go in favour of epilepsy.

Index

READER SUGGESTIONS SHEET

Please help us to improve the quality of our publications by completing and returning this sheet to us.

Author/Title: **The Art of History Taking** *By Kashinath Padhiary*

Your name and address:

Phone and Fax:

e-mail address:

How did you hear about this book? [please tick appropriate box (es)]

☐ Direct mail from publisher   ☐ Conference

☐ Bookshop   ☐ Book review

☐ Lecturer recommendation   ☐ Friends

☐ Other (please specify)   ☐ Website

Type of purchase: ☐ Direct purchase   ☐ Bookshop   ☐ Friends

Do you have any brief comments on the book?

Please return this sheet to the name and address given below.

JAYPEE BROTHERS
MEDICAL PUBLISHERS (P) LTD
EMCA House, 23/23B Ansari Road, Daryaganj
New Delhi 110 002, India

READER SUGGESTIONS SHEET

JAYPEE BROTHERS
MEDICAL PUBLISHERS (P) LTD